'This is an honest, sometimes brutally honest, account of Charlie Bacchus' experience of coping with MS and bipolar disorder. It is sometimes an uncomfortable read, sometimes hard to discern reality from fantasy, but always deeply personal, often funny, documenting exquisitely how the unconditional love of family and friends is so critical for survival in the face of a condition that robbed Charlie Bacchus of the future he anticipated. MS, and bipolar disorder, are often described as like being on a rollercoaster ride. Charlie Bacchus appears to have been on a monster of a ride, but with the love and honesty of family and friends, an absolute determination to accept who he is, and the opportunity to reflect deeply while writing this book, perhaps he is taming the two-headed monster that is MS and bipolar disorder.'

Prof Jonathan Evans, Professor of Applied Neuropsychology, University of Glasgow

'Inflicted by MS and bipolar disorder, Charlie tells the tale of living 25 years with these disorders, and how it affected his relationships, friends and family. With wonderful verve, we see him move from enthusiastic footballer and adventurous young rebel to facing the prospect of decline. This book will be of great interest to carers and patients alike.'

Michael Kopelman, Emeritus Professor of Neuropsychiatry, King's College London, UK

'This book provides an energetic and unfiltered perspective on life with a progressive neurological condition. Though the story is unique, its themes are of broad relevance: the importance of continuity in sense of identity (including sexual identity, which features conspicuously here), the appeal of storytelling in adapting to disability, the value of long-term relationships with coordinated health services, and above all the power of family resilience in living well with a neurological condition. I don't think you'll find another memoir quite like it, and recommend you have a read.'

Dr Jessica Fish, St George's University Hospitals NHS Trust & King's College London, UK

My Life with MS, Bipolar and Brain Injury

LIVING IN THE MOMENT

This is the remarkable story of Charlie Bacchus, who was diagnosed with a severe case of viral encephalitis and later with multiple sclerosis and bipolar. This moving, funny, sometimes explicit book charts his life, including recollections of his childhood, the acceptance of his diagnoses and his determination to carry on living to the full.

This book highlights many themes, such as the loss of independence and the challenges of hidden disabilities and visible differences. Although
This book highlights many themes, such as the loss of independence and the challenges of hidden disabilities and visible differences. Although the line between fantasy and reality is not always clear, Charlie's loving personality and hypomania allow him to maintain supportive connections and adapt to his situation.

Charlie's account provides support for patients who have brain injury and their families. This will be of great interest to professionals working in neurology, including occupational therapists, social workers and rehabilitation practitioners.

Charlie was first diagnosed with encephalitis, then multiple sclerosis and bipolar. He was an excellent footballer and believed in his career as a professional – when he realised he couldn't kick a ball anymore. Art and living life to the full became his passion.

Mab came to London to set up the French Music Office at the French Embassy. When she met Charlie, she was training to go back to psychology, her first vocation. Her private consultation as a French counselling psychologist is now thriving.

After Brain Injury: Survivor Stories

Series Editor: Barbara A. Wilson

This new series of books is aimed at those who have suffered a brain injury, and their families and carers. Each book focuses on a different condition, such as face blindness, amnesia and neglect, or diagnosis, such as encephalitis and locked-in syndrome, resulting from brain injury. Readers will learn about life before the brain injury, the early days of diagnosis, the effects of the brain injury, the process of rehabilitation, and life now. Alongside this personal perspective, professional commentary is also provided by a specialist in neuropsychological rehabilitation, making the books relevant for professionals working in rehabilitation such as psychologists, speech and language therapists, occupational therapists, social workers and rehabilitation doctors. They will also appeal to clinical psychology trainees and undergraduate and graduate students in neuropsychology, rehabilitation science, and related courses who value the case study approach.

With this series, we also hope to help expand awareness of brain injury and its consequences. The World Health Organisation has recently acknowledged the need to raise the profile of mental health issues (with the WHO Mental Health Action Plan 2013-20) and we believe there needs to be a similar focus on psychological, neurological and behavioural issues caused by brain disorder, and a deeper understanding of the importance of rehabilitation support. Giving a voice to these survivors of brain injury is a step in the right direction.

Published titles:

Rebuilding Life after Brain Injury
Dreamtalk
Sheena McDonald, Allan Little, Gail Robinson

Family Experience of Brain Injury
Surviving, Coping, Adjusting
Jo Clark-Wilson and Mark Holloway

For more information about this series, please visit: https://www.routledge.com/After-Brain-Injury-Survivor-Stories/book-series/ABI

My Life with MS, Bipolar and Brain Injury

LIVING IN THE MOMENT

By Charlie Bacchus

Facilitated by
Marie 'Mab' Beau

Routledge
Taylor & Francis Group
LONDON AND NEW YORK

First published 2020
by Routledge
2 Park Square, Milton Park, Abingdon, Oxon OX14 4RN

and by Routledge
52 Vanderbilt Avenue, New York, NY 10017

Routledge is an imprint of the Taylor & Francis Group, an informa business

British Library Cataloguing-in-Publication Data
A catalogue record for this book is available from the British Library

Library of Congress Cataloging-in-Publication Data
A catalog record has been requested for this book

ISBN: 978-1-138-33123-5 (hbk)
ISBN: 978-1-138-33128-0 (pbk)
ISBN: 978-0-429-44739-6 (ebk)

Typeset in Times New Roman
by Wearset Ltd, Boldon, Tyne and Wear

Contents

Foreword

I first met Charlie Bacchus in 1996, when, at the age of 19, he was admitted to our ward in a very elated and overactive state, characteristic of bipolar disorder. This soon settled and was followed by a more prolonged depression. Charlie had been diagnosed with multiple sclerosis (MS) about a year or so earlier, so this might have been a delayed psychological reaction to his illness. However, both elation and depression have commonly been noted in MS and are thought to be a direct consequence of the brain changes, although bipolar mood swings have been described less often.

Charlie experienced one more episode of acute elation, requiring hospital admission, again followed by a prolonged depression. However, after that, we managed to control his mood swings in an outpatient setting by manipulation of his medication, and by various psychological therapies, principally carried out by my excellent colleagues, clinical psychologists led by Dr Eli Jaldow and a counselling therapist, Ms Elisabeth Scott.

Charlie's charm and warmth were always evident at these outpatient meetings, and there was always a twinkle in his eye, especially when I was accompanied by an attractive female junior doctor, psychologist, trainee, or student. Also very evident, was the considerable support that Charlie derived from all his family, including both his parents, his sister and his brother. It has been sad to observe Charlie's physical decline, particularly in recent years, which he has borne with great stoicism and courage.

Much of this warmth and charm is evident in this book, and Charlie's personal assistant/ helper, Mab, has done a terrific job in eliciting Charlie's memories from him and getting them into print in such a coherent fashion. The book, it seems to me, falls into three parts.

The first part tells about Charlie's growing up, his football and the onset of his illness. I thought this was extremely well written, and it reminded me a bit of a book called *Brain on Fire* by Susannah Cahalan, a book on the experience of encephalitis, but there was even something of *Catcher in the Rye* about it. I leave the reader to decide whether or not this praise is overblown.

In the second part, we move more into Henry Miller/*Fifty Shades* territory. Charlie says at one point that his doctors knew all about his activities – well, not exactly! Some readers may wonder whether it is wise for Charlie to have revealed all this, and whether it is true. It is worth remembering that the white-matter changes in the frontal lobes of the brain (part of what happens in MS) do make people more disinhibited in what they say and do, and they can even make the boundary between reality and fantasy less clear (in an extreme form, there is what is called 'confabulation' of memories). Charlie says at one point in the book that he is not sure what was real and what was fantasy; but he has also said that this was the best part of his life, and he wants to have it included in this volume.

I thought that the third part of the book conveyed extremely well Charlie's more recent deterioration, the physical humiliations that this brings with it, as well as his sadness at the loss of his previous activities and relationships. I found this part very moving. Charlie is also extremely good on the ambiguities of the mother–son relationship, and how rightly proud he is of his mother.

In fact, Charlie's love for his family, and theirs for him, was evident throughout the book; and I witnessed this again at his fortieth birthday party at the end of last year. I take my hat off to all his splendid family, and to Mab who has put this book together so well, and particularly to Charlie himself and to Hannah ('the Motherhood'). In circumstances of family illness that would wear down or destroy the spirit of many other people, Hannah has fought magnificently for her family, and Charlie quite rightly conveys the warmth of their relationship.

Michael Kopelman, Emeritus Professor of Neuropsychiatry,
King's College London, based at St Thomas' Hospital

Preface

How this 'biovella' came to life

At the DASL (Disability Advice Service) offices, a charismatic young man in a wheelchair – a joking Jesus Christ lookalike – and his lovely mum welcomed me with a happy and warm smile. I was meeting them for a carer job interview. Right away, a wave of mutual empathy and sweet energy instilled this first shot of confidence that was much needed at that time. Charlie and Hannah asked very interesting well-prepared questions showing the depth of their reflection on their needs. Charlie was falling asleep one minute, joking and showing off the other, temporised by his mother and her unconditional love. I felt secured by her. So rare to feel that comfortable at a job interview! I had to restrain myself from joking back with Charlie.

A French-trained clinical psychologist, I was coming back to that sector after 30 years in the music industry and needed a job to get a foot into the British health system. I had dived into books, trainings and therapies myself. Moreover, I really needed to train my self-esteem.

My only question was for Charlie: 'Can you eventually stay alone at home?' 'Of course,' he said. 'Unfortunately not,' said Hannah. I was getting a better sense of their freedom and dependency issues.

My carer job started out by pushing Charlie around to coffee shops, to the park, to a reggae festival, and then to his art and printing lessons. It was OK but not very fulfilling and sometimes quite challenging – for instance, when he had to urgently pee in the bus using a bottle that I was not able to open, and then close. I had no idea this could happen just like that. I'm quite proud to have been able to deal with this quickly and calmly without anyone noticing!

The idea of writing his autobiography came about with Charlie's biggest fantasy: *The Silver-Tongued Cavalier*, the film about his life that he was so proud to tell everyone about. Until recently, he enjoyed offering loads of strangers – especially nice girls and ladies – a role in the movie. It was a great way to start a conversation with ladies.

I had not heard about narrative therapy yet, but it was obvious that Charlie needed:

- to be heard and recognised, eventually as an exceptional, talented and intelligent person
- to make sense and use of many fantastic experiences and memories, especially his loving and positive thinking abilities
- to grieve his football champion status as well as many other issues such as body agility and ability, independence, sex, marriage and building a family.

It was also promising to be a funny and intelligent piece of live research on resilience, mental health, MS, drugs and sex, and more.

Not only has my offer to write his story been very welcome but it was easy to kick off, as Charlie had already rehearsed and/or performed the first sentences to as many people as possible. Suddenly, he didn't have to impose himself on strangers or uninterested people; he was actually making it happen, he was diving into it, being questioned about himself and his amazing life, having fun and making me laugh a lot and shout as well.

It was not easy for me to accept and work with:

- his uncontrolled attention deficit: while we work, he needs to touch everything around him, especially his phone. He sometimes had to make an effort to switch off the TV while working, or to not check his lottery tickets
- his narrative style and abilities. He would sometimes repeat the same things over and over – which may also be apparent in the book. Typical Charlie! He would start every sentence about anyone with 'X is an amazing person' or 'Our souls connected right away', and would often stop there. It is hard for him to access his memory or his internal glossary so I really had to delve deeply into his brain. I often had the impression he was just lazy, waiting for me to bring his life back to him. I sometimes felt I was doing most of the work and he was just approving or not, rephrasing it in better English. Therefore, I had to constantly make sure I was not influencing, projecting or interpreting, although I certainly did. But then Hannah's input and referencing

were always useful. We have reread and edited together quite a few times

- the interpretation of his fantasies as real truth. Charlie believes in his dreams so it is sometimes difficult to discover the true reality of some of his stories. However, I believe it is his own truth anyway. His perception, feelings and interpretation are real, even if troubled by illness or just by frustration. When doubting too much or having his mum denying some facts and stories, I would insist on finding out the truth. Sometimes he would kindly admit it was just a fantasy, sometimes he would stick so hard to his version that we would decide to keep it and just mention the idea that it may be a fantasy felt as reality. Sometimes it was really difficult to find out, as he would easily change his mind according to the way I was questioning him, to his mood or his inclination to please or to dream … Therefore I sometimes had to dig really hard, but then, as he would always tend to agree and be positive, he would easily accept my interpretation. So, I would leave it for another time and go back to it later, trying to grasp the core of his feelings. It would always bring us to some interesting insights and we would clinch an understanding of his experience.

About the title: Charlie was clearly passionate about *The Silver-Tongued Cavalier*. This title had been official for about two years, until it seemed obvious that it was limiting him to his oral abilities when the book had so much more to say about him. When we started writing, Charlie was at the difficult stage where he had to come to terms with the loss of his sex-god status. After grieving his football champion status, he had to let go of his sexual prowess. Sex was one of his most favourite subjects. I believe that talking about sex with a middle-aged French woman and writing down all his adventures helped him to make sense of them. Actually, he does not talk about it as much anymore. I was happy to rationally explain to him a few things that he thought were his sole privilege. Whether some were definitely true or just a fantasy, we both believe that these kinky stories would 'keep the book live and well' (quoting Charlie) and make it more attractive to the public. Moreover, they were indeed one of the most important parts of his life. We can all understand how difficult it must have been for his mum to read them and accept they would eventually be published.

About the people: it has been hard to convince Charlie to be cautious about the relationships he is talking about in his book. His free spirit would not see why it might make them feel very uncomfortable and put them in a difficult position. I must thank Hannah for her constant care to make sure nobody gets hurt and to protect Charlie from his own unique challenges. It has not always been easy for me to accept what I call British political correctness, which needs to avoid mentioning some real negative feelings and dilutes them into something less tangible and more acceptable. Don't get me wrong; I do appreciate very much its positive effects as well, as I learnt to be tolerant and a lot less judgemental – especially as Charlie is totally accepting and makes fun of his own kind of craziness, which is one of his numerous charms.

The writing process started in June 2012 and we finished the first editing work in July 2016. We first worked for a couple of hours twice a week, then only once a week and finally once every fortnight, as my own work kicked off really strongly (partly thanks to the confidence given me by Charlie). Those last three years saw some dramatic changes in Charlie's life: no more sex, no more drugs or even cigarette addiction; no use of his legs; protective pads; no chance of having a so-called independent life without support, on his own away from his parents' home, nor even at home. Charlie speaks in the present tense, so the reader sees the changes happening as the book goes along. We intended to keep things chronological, but the chronology doesn't fit with every chapter or with the way Charlie remembers things.

I really didn't mind the fact that he would fall asleep for a few minutes, go to the toilet quite often, ask for music to be played (he likes any kind of music and enjoyed very much my own favourite styles). But my Latin temper would often show some impatience. As a matter of fact, Charlie helped me a lot to work on that. In concentrating on him, I managed to overcome that really bad habit and discovered I could be patient and tolerant. Whew! What a fantastic training for me as a reborn psychologist! I also had to put down some strict limits and express my own needs clearly. Most of the time, it was just a warm, joyful, rich exchange. The slowest sessions may have come up with just a couple of paragraphs, but always with an amazing way of saying things. Charlie would naturally be empathetic, asking about my close ones, always remembering to care about my own well-being, always telling me he loves me. This relationship, starting as a small job, quickly became a process of strong mutual encouragement thanks to its creative and very personal aspects.

Charlie gave me the greatest mindfulness lesson ever, much better than in any book or training session, or even a meeting with the Dalai Lama. Additionally, both Charlie and his mum helped me a lot with my own confidence, which was one of my main issues when I started working with them: confidence in my ability to deal with other people's pain, confidence to fit into the British system and language, confidence in my previous training in psychopathology, confidence in my own self.

It is absolutely amazing to see how Charlie's mental state is helping him to cope with his neurological and physical issues.

It is only now that the book is finished and my own career as a counselling psychologist is thriving that I realise that I never ever intended to bring Charlie any kind of counselling, therapy or psychoeducation. I was just interested in his story, the telling of which was, in itself, the best way for him to face his situation. Anyway, given his personality, we believe that Charlie would not have accepted another approach.

Most striking is Charlie's happy, kind and loving character, showing how love has no limits and helping him to deal with many tough situations by keeping on enjoying life in the present moment.

MAB

Chapter 1

The rise and fall of a football star

I was already kicking hard in the womb. The little Scorpio Fire Dragon was born splashing blood all over the hospital's birthing room. It seems that right from the start I was alive and kicking in all the manners of the expression, as well as determined to leave a mark.

Early in primary school I kept on kicking a tennis ball and it quickly became a passion. It really helped me hone my skills for football, as the bigger ball appeared a lot easier to play around with. Unfortunately, my brother Matt has always hated football, just like any other sport, so I always wanted to go out and play on the Common with other kids. My parents – as protective as most – would not let me go there alone, so they got me into the Little League team when I was about seven. I quickly became a striker and that's what I have always been, running in front, controlling the ball and banging it into the back of the net. It felt completely natural and easy, as my legs and feet were so fast and interlinked, my eyes were everywhere and my mental ability was completely locked on the game. I loved that so much.

When I was ten, the manager of a South London team spotted me playing on the Common and offered me the chance to come and play in the next cup match in the team called Accra (like the capital in Ghana, West Africa). It was the team of a daunting estate with a rough reputation. I arrived for the quarter-final match and didn't mind being the only white boy. The speed of the game was quite different from playing with the Little League team. It was energising and raised my game. In the second half of the match, we were five nil down so I decided to initiate my magic boots and scored a double hat trick (six goals). The boys were so surprised, they were sucking their teeth and wouldn't express any compliments, but I could feel their respect as I'd kept them in the cup.

Expectations were high for the semi-final and the atmosphere was really different. The heat was on, and the pressure was especially on me as I'd scored a double hat trick in the quarters. The guys were all playing it rough – it wasn't a pure game anymore but a battle. Moreover, the football field was on a big hill, which was bizarre and difficult to play on, as I was used to the Common, which is the flattest common in the world to me. I was definitely not feeling as comfortable as usual in my striker boots that day and I didn't score, although I had a couple of opportunities. I could hear teeth being sucked around when I was missing the goals. It was a shock-horror for me, as we ended up losing one nil on that semi-final stage.

To cheer ourselves up a bit, I and one of the boys in the team went to buy a chocolate bar at the local shop on the estate. A strange guy in the shop gave me a killer look, staring right at me with hate and resentment and just spat at me, 'I'm gonna fuckin kill you!' I couldn't comprehend his raging at me. I was too young to understand that he was on some kind of heavy drug, probably crack, and that it was a race-and-class issue. I was paralysed by this moment. Fortunately, the shop manager obviously knew this guy and quietened him down right away. So, it appeared he was not that dangerous, but I felt scared enough to tell my parents about it. They explained to me about the problems and violence that were occurring on those estates and decided not to let me go back to play with that team again. That was my first experience of danger and the complexities of racism and class discrimination.

It would be fair to say that it was a time when competitive sports were not acceptable in the state system and so football wasn't being played in those schools. Because of my football ability my father especially wanted me to have the opportunity to continue to improve. My parents were not in agreement about private school education, and had to have counselling to come to an agreement. The compromise was an independent day school, which was, at that time, like a fee-paying grammar school. I would be safe and happy to play football a lot in its beautiful grounds and develop all kind of other abilities and talents, especially in the arts, as well as good opportunities for socialising. I've heard since then that this exemplary school's founder put his money into education for poor kids and orphans to show his good values and will.

At school, I fell deeply in love for the first time. I was 16 years old, and that cutie pie was taking the same bus as me. She was four years younger. Being around her was making me feel so happy. She was a perfect blonde beauty, a very young version of Pamela Anderson without the boob job, who easily managed to wake up my first hormonal feelings. I enjoyed talking to her, discovering completely new sensations and feeling my willy waking up. I was also enticed by the fact that she was attracted to me as well. That was giving me a new kind of pride and making me feel frenzied. I was discovering my own charms. The whole thing was a new sensation, I was convinced it was pure love, or was it just lust and teenage hormones? I was quite naive about sexual feelings as I had reached puberty quite late at 15. Sex was not something we would talk about frequently at home. We were warned about AIDS though. I had experienced only one wank, fantasising about one of my parents' friends who in my eyes had the most glorious breasts.

Anyway, that young cutie awakened sexual feelings in me even though we never even kissed. First, because I was more obsessed with football. Second, my schoolmates were laughing at me hanging around such a young girl, calling me a paedophile. I found myself happy with a platonic bus-ride love. We managed to build a nice friendship and kept in touch on the phone. She felt very concerned when she learnt I was unwell a few years later and came to visit me in hospital. I hadn't seen her for ages. She was looking incredible and told me, among other things, that she had worked as a stripper during the holidays. This made me fantasise about rushing to the toilets with her for some kinky games but the recollection of our first platonic love remained and kept our relationship pure. However, she never got back in touch after that visit.

Back to my early football passion. I always loved how football flows: when you have a good defence, the ball is easily fed forward to the middle field and then on to the strikers and into the net. The team effort and unity really got me going. The glory of a victory was the success of that teamwork as well as my own personal triumph. When me and my best mate, who was the best defender, went to the trials for Senior League we got in immediately. As an excellent striker I was often in the limelight. My confidence was living on a high. I was following my dad as a big supporter of the Spurs and we were regularly going to White Hart Lane in Tottenham. I was inspired by Hoddle and Woddle doing their tricks on the pitch. It was such a special time with my father, not only belonging to a vibrant group of men but also growing close to my dad. Football was definitely the most exciting thing in my life.

I played for lots of brilliant football teams in London. When I was 17, a professional coach said I could become a professional footballer and may play for England. This, added to my good looks and my special way with the ladies, was arousing some jealousy. I was accepting this as the other side of the coin and was enjoying my life to the maximum.

While I was at school in sixth form doing A levels, something pretty bad struck my life. It all started in the mouth. I thought I had a mouth ulcer because my left bottom jaw was very dull. My little finger on the left hand was getting numb and then my fingers followed suit. Within a week, my little left toe, my left arm and the whole left part of my body, including my left ball and left-hand side of my penis!!! My leg went to sleep altogether, with my left eye as well. I was also vomiting profusely. I was diagnosed with viral encephalitis and stayed in hospital for a month or so for further examinations and treatments. The damage of the encephalitis was spreading. The neurologist gave me high doses of steroids, which quickly helped ease the inflammation and pumped me up physically and mentally. It was probably the first time I got really high and at the same time felt healthy again. This may have triggered some future drug inclination. The doctor said I would be back playing football within six months but in fact the infection was already in my brain. I don't know how much those steroids may have also triggered other complications.

During that first stay in hospital I was so excited I remember trying to climb up onto the window ledges to embrace the beautiful view of the Houses of Parliament. I felt both imprisoned and invincible at the same time. This strange feeling and behaviour have never left me since. I would never have guessed that being trapped and happy at the same time would be my fate or is it just my lifetime journey? At least my positive mental attitude is still helping me to cope with the entrapment. I realise that this attitude is at the same time protecting me and also probably spearheading my feeling of immunity. Since that first time in hospital, I have had the feeling that my illness is playing tricks on me.

Stuck in hospital, my spontaneous reaction was to draw. I was drawing everything, from the Houses of Parliament out of the window to the people in my ward, which was the cancer ward. I could feel suffering and death all around me. Not only time-consuming, drawing was a great way to get closer to people and share experiences and ailments, as I was talking to them whilst I drew. It was quite liberating and intriguing to get deeper and deeper into other people's psyches and into my own inner feelings. It was quite an invigorating experience even though these people knew that they were coming to the final days of their lives. Alongside this, I also had loads of friends and family visiting every day. We all wanted to believe the doctor's reassuring words.

Out of hospital, I was so happy to be able to strike the ball again in the back of the net as I used to do all the time. However, at school my behaviour was becoming a bit disruptive, particularly in my art class. I had already reached puberty but all my energy had been concentrated onto the football field. Suddenly now, my sexuality awakened. I was starting to have great fantasies and was feeling really excited and happy all the time, so happy that it was not real. As a matter of fact, I was still at the age where the front cortex is developing and both this wicked virus and those steroids had an effect on my brain, opening up some new neurones and kicking in mania and sometimes depression, bringing me to this unfortunate but magical mental trip and confusion. Was it the virus or the steroids? Probably both. Who knows?

Thanks to the heavy steroid treatments, the numb feelings on the left side had totally disappeared, but something else happened. The new disaster struck during the summer holiday as the whole family was travelling to Norway to visit my godfather. All my mates had succeeded in their A levels, finished with school and were off to party in South Africa. I had to stay with my family for the summer as I needed rest and supervision in a convalescent state of mind. Because of all the time spent in hospital, my only plan was to go back to school in September to do my A levels again. I was 'nough pissed off indeed!

We were going to visit my godfather in Norway and had taken the ferry across from Newcastle. While in the car I started puking so much that it reminded us of the first symptoms of what we had thought was encephalitis. We got so frightened that I was taken to a Norwegian hospital. The only thing I can now clearly remember is the dazzling and beautiful Norwegian nurses. Their blondness, freshness and healthiness, together with their huge breasts and soft touches. Although I was very scared, at a time when my hormones were being awakened, my memories are still of an exciting and happy experience. After five days, the Norwegian doctor diagnosed multiple sclerosis (MS).

Conflictingly, on our return to England, my English consultant continued to be unsure about the MS diagnosis. We went to have a second opinion at the National Centre for Neurological Illness in London as to what drugs I should take. The consultant there didn't deny MS but suggested we wait until research for MS treatments was more advanced. They also preferred to see how the illness developed. I was really young to get an MS diagnosis and they didn't want to take more unnecessary risks with my health.

I could feel all this indecision, and thought these experts were afraid to talk with me about my neurological condition and its possible complications. My mum, who had been a nurse, had the balls to tell me clearly about the illness. She did this with all her love and commitment and I knew she would take care of me and support me unconditionally. I was almost 18, an age when I was supposedly able to take some responsibilities for myself. Knowing about the illness and its potential seriousness should have helped me take it more seriously, should have helped me become careful, to treat myself properly in order to keep my nerves and neurones safe and healthy, to try to avoid the danger of developing too quickly.

In contrast, I was just becoming an angry frustrated teenager feeling that death was around the corner. As a survival reflex, I started rejecting everything that was happening to me and around me. I was fighting against what was happening to me. I was 'stuck' being a troubled kid rather than a young adult facing a heavy challenge. That is when and why I started living in denial.

Back to London and into the sixth form, I went back to the football field but quickly realised I didn't quite have the touch I used to have. Something huge was missing: the natural cohesion and speed between my mind and my body had disappeared. What had happened to my legs? I couldn't believe it and carried on trying to catch back what had been stolen from me. But I didn't even dare go back to playing with a team. The Charlie Bacchus without sport was not the me I used to know. The only thing I knew was that my great passion for football had changed its route, my reason for life was dying away. The illness would strongly affect my nerves and I would be under heavy treatment, not knowing anything about the consequences.

One of the main aspects of MS is that it develops completely differently from one person to another – nothing can be planned. However, we do know that looking after yourself and the nerves is the most important thing to keep the illness at bay. Any strong challenge to the brain can be really damaging. I was 17 and a half, totally confused and cut up, as I couldn't figure out my life without football. I'd been the best striker on the field and now I was nobody. Maybe I'd been too lucky and hadn't deserved so much success. I had never been depressed before. Sometimes I was definitely feeling very lost and angry – never angry at anyone though, just angry at the fact I could not enjoy my passion and be number one on the field. In class, especially in art, I was quite disruptive, needing to express my frustration and be noticed as well. The teacher had difficulty in accepting my behaviour and I was regularly ejected from the class. I understand now that this behaviour was also due to the inflammation and scarring of my frontal lobe.

Fortunately, the sadness would never last; deep inside I still trusted life thanks to my family's beautiful soul-affirming attitude. Thanks to my amazing parent's unconditional love and wise words, my family understood me and gave me even more inner strength. I was feeling safe and loved, and I knew they would all be right there for me, including the extended family and friends. I could feel they were very upset but most importantly they were all standing right by me. Despite, or because of, those low places where my mind would take me, I was entering a new realm full of love and understanding. I had been brought up in the awareness that caring, loving and being creative can bring more joy and strength than physical abilities and social success. I don't know exactly how she did it, but my mum gave me an even higher sense of this by encouraging me to develop my loving and creative ways. That is how my heart dived into ART in a big way. Here is an extract of an essay written for my A level in Art showing how the bipolarity was already striking before anyone had mentioned it.

Transfixed by moments in time

The reason why I have chosen to do this subject is because I feel I can strongly relate to the 'frozen moments in time'. Last May my world was full. Full of things which anyone of my age would be doing at any moment in time. I was a keen sportsman, and in particular I loved football. I could say that it was the love of my life. I thought that I had a mouth ulcer, because my left bottom jaw was very numb. Various check-ups occurred, and within two weeks my whole body was numb. I couldn't see, I couldn't stop throwing up and I was put on a large dose of steroids. I was scared, angry, out of control, over the top, invincible. They called it viral encephalitis. It changed my life, temporally, so I thought, because you do recover from viral encephalitis. Relapses continued throughout the year, making it difficult to concentrate and to continue with my subjects as well as I had hoped. Last September, while in hospital in Norway, I was diagnosed with multiple sclerosis.... Frozen moment in time ... and so many other frozen moments in time since then. This was my initial reaction to the question. But then how could I invest with narrative power, within my painting, the story of these past months. I felt it was important to explore the artists mentioned in the question alongside the artist Egon Schiele, who I feel has great capacity to explore human depths.

The painting I have chosen to do is the story of two sides of a personality. Two people in one, with different emotions and different stories to tell. The picture of myself on the left is the invincible me – my understanding of myself when I am over the top, the side of me which believes that I can do anything I want, the me that needs no fear, the me that people find difficult. The me that is full of fun, the me that can rule ... that can rule the world, the me that needs not to conform. They call it a euphoric state. The other portrait is the other side of me, a change that can happen overnight or within an hour, the me that can draw and begin to paint one of my preparation portraits, the angry masked face, and then not be able to finish it. This change – this depression – happened during my art exam, when despair and anxiety took over, changing my mood, two sides of a personality. As Kitaj said: 'My idea of art is that it conceals and reveals one's life, and that what it confesses is as Kafka called it a "rumour of true things".'

I am at the beginning of a journey, but what I have learnt by myself, and alongside other people who meant a lot to me, is that each experience that any one of us has in the space of time is a frozen moment in time, and that the way we deal with any situation is dependent upon what we have experienced before it has occurred. I've reached the same level as Egon Schiele in 'coming to terms with death in the midst of life, which makes your mind so much freer'.

More than 20 years later, I still feel that my life is a frozen moment in time. However, I have come to terms with the depressive moments and I have truly lived my life to the full, so full that I have damaged my neurologic system even more. Obviously, I was so scared of that frozen life in front of me that I challenged it with hubristic and fierce fun. It is definitely now that I am 'coming to terms with death in the midst of life', when my body is getting worse and my mind feels freer thanks to this new narrative power of the autobiography. Making my point on the page may seem to freeze it on the computer screen, but more importantly it does untrap it from my mind, and the words that can be read by other people give it life.

Losing my virginity

At the time of doing my A levels, I was discovering my illness and throwing myself into creativity.

I was ready to explore the female form. Before MS, I was so obsessed with my football career that I didn't think about romance. Getting the ball into the net was far more natural and easier than getting my dick into a girl's pussy. But the steroids may also have played their part. I had met my first girlfriend at school and we were really good friends. She was very arty, bubbly and cute. We could talk about anything and she was upset by my new challenge. We were not in love but our hormones drew us to each other, we felt physically attracted and it was time to discover this delectable adult part of life.

On that Friday evening, we had a few drinks at a friend's, which probably helped us to feel that special sexual connection and decided to go back to my house. I asked my dad if he had a condom. He said with a knowing smile, 'You're lucky, I've got one left', and then we went to my room, had a couple of drinks and the gates were opening. I softly took her clothes off, needing her help for the bra (of course that was something I had never come across on a football field), discovering with loads of joy and excitement her beautiful curves and, for the first time in my life, breasts and their nipples. I played around with them first like they were Star Wars toys and very quickly my mouth and tongue were urged on to a discovery trip in this new galaxy. She was obviously enjoying it very much, bubbling out some sounds of excitement that I had never heard before and that made my cock feel like the Millennium Falcon.

My erection was so hard that my penis rocket went directly into its new tropical territory, slid in neatly into that warm and wet treasure box. It was such a beautiful thing to have my phallus discovering a woman's intimacy. We knew each other so well and felt so comfortable in each other's company that it felt very natural and fun. It was a breakthrough into a new glorious playground with brand new sensations, sights, smells and sounds. Amazing to watch her eyes getting crazy, her cheeks getting *rouge*, her whole body tensing, trembling and firing up. She had several huge orgasms. I was not expecting my penis to provoke that kind of tremor and was feeling extremely proud. Losing my virginity was like sliding effortlessly up Mount Everest, or scoring a goal and exhilarating a whole team of players and their supporters. Discovering that I could easily bring a lady to that level of joy gave me great confidence for the future ahead.

However, I was a bit surprised to have such a hard-on, lasting all night – but I couldn't come! I finally wanked off in front of her, watching my phallus exploding three metres up to the lights on the ceiling. My first orgasm with a lady made me feel extremely fulfilled about my existence on this planet, grateful to the universe. Now it was like doing a little jig on top of Everest, or as if I had scored a triple hat-trick. I finally felt back on top of the world and was entering a new amazing ground for me to play on – this was my ultimate league.

I quickly fell in love with sex, helped by my joyful, smiley looks, good body, education and wit. It quickly became an addiction, even though, or because, I couldn't come inside a woman. Indeed, that first ejaculation was not only ground-breaking but it happened to be one of the only orgasms I have ever sensed. That mystery has still not been solved 20 years later, but at least it naturally taught me the splendour of love through Tantric sex. Before we get into my naughty and glorious sexual history, it is important to talk about my family, as they are the strongest and deepest roots of my confidence and my loving existence.

Chapter 2

My free-spirited family

I was very fortunate to be born to a great family in London. We live in a very lively area, buzzing with young people coming to have fun almost every evening of the week. I guess people enjoy it because of its historical buildings and the Common that gives it a kind of homely and relaxed feel. The Common is known as a free-spirited huge meadow where anyone can do anything (and I have done so much there …). People living here are both affluent and multicultural. Loads of students and young people also live here, a university halls of residence used to be situated here. It is becoming very gentrified, attracting people from all over the world. The area where I live is quiet, and is becoming very affluent now. Back in history there were people who came from here who actively campaigned for the abolition of slavery and for other reforms such as ones about child labour and prison. They also set up charities in the British colonies. This kind of social activist mind-set is close to my family's culture and I like to consider myself as a generous and open-minded individual. This attitude towards life has taken me to many dazzling and insane places and has taught me many lessons.

When my parents moved in, the area had completely changed into an unsafe hood. Ironically, the affluent people who made their money in the colonies left, to be replaced by the people who'd been colonised. Loads of black people came in the 50s as part of the post-war immigration boom. Estates were built among the mansions and because of little and no investment in the estates the area became quite dejected and unsafe. When I was a child, the place was even more multicultural than now, which I really loved. I never ever felt unsafe, certainly because my family was never threatened, and also probably because of my loving personality.

I really enjoy living here, blessed with beauty, love and joy, as well as peace and wisdom coming from all over the world and needing all these centuries to build up. I am so fortunate to live in this place and space. I am glad to have skipped so many areas of violence. Diplomacy and democracy have come such a long way. However, democracy, especially, is no guarantee against violence anymore. It seems that capitalism and wonga (money) make the world just as violent as before, hiding behind corruption, new technologies and fake smiles. I cannot tell you how much I fervently dislike fake smiles. Hubris – arrogant pride against the gods – is still the main power anyway. I can feel it inside me as well. I am not really proud of it but it's always been there, helping me to conquer my inner fear of the future.

Actually, I would rather believe in the mutual nurturing of self-power and the glory of love. If you can link both, you are on to a winner. Actions in the name of love can only return in a good way. I have been brought up in the belief that if you act well in life, with love, caring and sharing, nothing bad within your soul can happen to you. I believe in family love which should go far beyond all kind of internal squabbles.

My brother, my hero

I am so happy to introduce everyone to my biggest hero and best protector, my brother Matt. I love him more than anyone could ever love! He knows how to dance very very well and he is an actor. He had a role as a lunatic in *Quills*, the movie about the last days of the Marquis de Sade, and fell in love with the main actress Kate Winslet. So now Matt wants to drink champagne all the time and likes to think he would do it in Hollywood. He has always been obsessed by soap operas and musicals (which give another dimension to soaps). He receives a soap mag every week and knows everything that's going on. Even though he cannot read or write very well, he's running his own soap mag with all the pictures and stories he's collecting. He uses glue stick and scissors to create his own page-design style. Actually, he did produce his own soap performance with his good friend Matt B. who is a brilliant actor and director. The play was called *Matt Matt the Opera* – he was the superstar and had seven fiancées, including Kate Winslet who was stalking him, and he was living between New York and California in the largest penthouses known to the world. This play has been performed a few times at the local arts centre. It was so incredible and dazzling that it was meant to be played at the Edinburgh festival, but the money was not there. Matt was not even disappointed because he is never frustrated, always the happiest in the house. Whatever is on TV, he is tuned in and repeats everything the actors say, as if he'd written the soap and had been the most focussed director. He uses and talks to a particular old trainer as a link between himself and the characters in the soaps and as a tool to communicate with the actors. When he goes to the cinema or theatre, he knows how to behave, shutting up and listening. Even though he's very sociable, I really wonder what he would do if there wasn't a single TV in the world.

Matt is also artistic. Matt is my minder in a big way. He is always on my side, even though we're very competitive. Our brother rivalry is more of a joy than a hindrance, because it helps us to go forward and we easily agree and find out what is best for each of us. He's trying to steal my best girlfriends, but I don't mind because I know he won't get them in the end. He's a great judge of the girls and knows if one is good enough for me. He always knows when something is wrong or right. He would strongly criticise me if I was flirting with someone and might be on the verge of cheating on somebody.

Matt is always happy

Matt is a person with a learning disability, but I can see he is more intelligent than most as he can tell immediately about people's souls. Without being able to tell why, he knows right away what is good or bad for me – much better than I can – and manages to stop me going in the wrong direction. I believe I'm very sensitive but he is a lot more sensitive in many many ways.

Matt works really hard at the local arts centre, in the café and in the kitchen, producing lunches. He's a legend there –he's filling up the place with his good vibes. Having Matt as a brother taught me how to love. I feel everyone should have a child like Matt in their family to understand what unconditional love is all about. I feel so safe with my brother; I know he will always look after me. And he knows I will always look after him. I have such an amazing family around me. I really don't know how I would have coped with MS and bipolar and various events if they hadn't been there.

When Matt was born Mum and Dad came back from the hospital with him and told us our brother was a bit different. My sister and I said in unison, 'We don't care, he's our brother', and it's always been that way since. We love him with all our hearts and will always protect him.

When we were young children and went out to the shop, loads of people would stare at him'; therefore I felt I had to gently tell them, 'This is my brother, there's nothing wrong with him, he's fantastic, please don't stare at him'. So they would feel sorry, smile at my dazzling looks but still wouldn't dare talk to him. It was like I was an angel and he was a devil. It really hurt me. What an awful weird feeling to have regularly from an early age! I wasn't angry, because I'm never angry anyway, but I was extremely upset with the unfairness of the world. The pain was such that it may have had an impact on my brain. I knew Matt was aware and suffering from being different and being stared at. I wouldn't even mention these shockers to my parents to avoid them having more pain.

I was Matt's protector. Now he is my own protector and people are staring at me instead of him. Matt is the boss now. He can be very controlling, more than Mum, and becomes quite nervous about me breaking the limits, especially on money. I truly appreciate when Matt is my gentle carer, especially when I need him to push me around in my wheelchair. Matt's values are very strong and he sticks to them with loyalty, when I would rather pick and choose among my own vast array of principles. Bipolar easily throws any morals and principles out of the window. Matt can be indignant towards me. He easily picks on my neurotic oral habits. He hates when I'm sucking and chewing things, probably because he has a chewing-gum phobia. He also hates when I talk to people on the street.

His intelligence is different, in the sanest possible way: he doesn't care about how the world is running, he doesn't care about things that are totally out of his control but he is aware of everything that happens around him. He can feel any little tension, and he will express his feelings if this can help ease the situation or he will just leave the place. You can tell from his face if there is anything going wrong for him or for the people he loves.

Matt has such fantastic friends. They are all good people who can see his brilliance. Matt has had two girlfriends and he respects them and himself so much.

My brother has the most amazing memory; he reminds me of when I had a photographic memory. I *could* be jealous, but no, the love is so strong that I don't get too jealous, I'm just proud. Matt loves to have his back scratched and I like to be there for him and scratch his back for a few minutes. I can make him laugh loud in tickling the lower part of his back, though he doesn't purr.

I feel so lucky to have Matt as a brother; his beautiful smile and his energy spread joy everywhere he goes.

Flying safe with grandparents

My grandparents were brilliant people with a lot of kick. Both couples were based in Africa and were particularly open-minded for their time. They were crucial for my growth, as they would let me fly in a contained manner. Both couples got on really well and chose to end their life journey in the home counties where we spent all our childhood weekends and most holidays.

The grandparents I built the closest relationship with were my mother's parents. I was really proud of my grandfather; he had achieved so much in the army. He served in Burma against the Japanese during the Second World War. He was such a strong and soft character and a brilliant man that everyone respected and loved. He was my rock, bringing order to my life and eventually became my chief army consultant for my games.

I really enjoyed going out for walks with him and the dog Raffles. Raffles used to be our own dog. As a golden retriever, he needed space and therefore we gave him to my grandparents in the country where he could be free to run in the copse. I was very sad when he left our house, but I knew he would be much happier and was not exiting my life. Actually, this was even better for both my grandfather and Raffles, as they built a very special bond. They were as close as Hannibal and his elephants, listening to and trusting each other unconditionally. It looked even deeper and stronger than a human relationship. When Grandfather B passed away, Raffles was so sad that his spirit left him and he slowly retired from life.

He was not the only animal to befriend Grandfather B: there was a deer that we would regularly meet during our walks. When we were crossing his territory, he would recognise us and pop his head up out of the bushes. He was obviously leaving his family to come and say hello, just making sure we'd seen him. Actually we saw him grow up. I felt that deer was also my friend and he was making those walks even more special. After Grandfather B's funeral we all went up into the wood to leave a flowered wreath and Mum planted a tree as a homage to her dad. A few days later I asked Mum if I could stay up in the wood to remember him. It was in this very quiet and beautiful place that the deer appeared to me in all its beauty and strength. I didn't know then that it was the last time I'd see him. I felt he came to share Grandfather B's memory with me and Raffles.

A few months later I was missing Grandfather B so much, I took Raffles for a walk and to pay a visit to his tree, and there it was: the deer had passed away as well, after Grandfather B died and by his tree. Raffles gave him a good smell and didn't dare pee on him. I knew he recognised him. We were both touched by this mark of affection to my granddad. I decided to rename the deer Hercules, because he was as forceful and strong as my grandfather, and to take the time to bury him. I had learnt about digging big holes while I was at Woodcraft Folk and went to get Grandfather B's tools. It took me an afternoon, and Raffles was there with me for our little ceremony. I just made up a prayer for both my grandfather and the deer. Some people think this whole story about the deer is a fantasy but to me it is as real and powerful as the sun.

Grandfather B was a great role model, guiding me about being a good man respecting everyone, including the bad people and those who are different from us. As a matter of fact, my basic education from home was all about respect – so much respect that they didn't manage to teach me to stay away from bad people.

Grandfather B was killed by his smoking habit. Both he and my grandmother were very heavy smokers and I got this really bad habit from them. How could I fight an addiction archetyped by my role models? I became a chainsmoker, aware that I am facing the same kind of death as my dear grandparents, even though it was so painful to see Grandfather B suffering from lung cancer. His death was certainly the worst moment of my childhood. I know I will be confronted with that same finale, just a bit quicker and harder than the majority of people. However, I feel that my life has been stolen from me already, crucifying me. Therefore earlier pain and death does not mean much. In a way I am accelerating my ill condition and life conclusion by smoking like a lunatic, as well as taking part in other frowned-upon and dangerous endeavours. As I feel my life is drifting away, I am smoking it away as if each puff was the last, sucking on the butt so hard that the cigarette is being consumed very fast, consuming my index finger my money and my health as well.

I like to believe that Granny B gave me my first cigarette when I was about 15. I knew from my grandfather's death and my parents' advice that it was very dangerous, therefore I asked Granny B why she kept on smoking. She softly answered with a cheeky smile: 'Try for yourself'. It was a great way to rebel against my parents and life's boundaries with the encouragement of the classy older lady in my life.

Granny B survived her husband for a few years and came to live around the corner from us. I was always so close to her and we got on really well. We connected in a true spiritual fashion. As soon as we saw each other our hearts were warmed. I could tell her confidential things that she would keep secret, which taught me how trust is important in life. It's so helpful and valuable to be able to safely release things you couldn't tell your parents and to be understood and cared for by such an amazing lady like my grandmother. It's like having a ball played through to me on the football field, when other people's trust and my own self-confidence gave me security to fly around with the ball and rarely miss the goal. Even if I'd miss it once in a while, it would not be a problem because I knew I'd score next time.

In the same way, I was feeling completely free, balanced and secure with Granny B, full of confidence and belief in life and myself. Approaching the end of her life, she freed herself even more and was always careful to keep her independence, although respecting other people's ways. I used to take around Sunday lunch for both of us and we would watch Poirot together. (Now because of my illness I cannot even carry a plate around the kitchen.) Although she looked very classy to me, Granny B could be a really good swearer. One day when my mum insisted she came to us for Sunday lunch, my father went to collect her and said, 'Come on Granny B, look it's a beautiful day', and she retorted 'FUCK THE DAY'. How many people would like to say this at times in life? It needs just a bit of sensitivity and maturity to know where and when to do that. It also taught me about freedom and self-control. Unfortunately she died when I was 15, just before I entered the realms of illness, madness and ladies.

I was on holiday in Sweden when she passed away and couldn't be with her, holding her hand and saying goodbye. I wish she had lived forever. Nevertheless, she is still there in my psyche, supporting me with deep love. I know she is around me somewhere; even if she is only in my own thoughts, she still brings me complete security. When I have a difficult decision to make, I can feel her soul and spirit with me, giving me some solid guidance. Sadly, she is not there to advice me with my relationships. I could well have been married with children if she had been around to teach me things about women. Her love is still there, giving me that confidence to go on with my existence.

My father's father, Grandfather D, was born in the Far East and spent most of his life in East Africa. He was a strong-in-spirit man. My great-grandfather was killed in the First World War when Grandfather D was very young. He refused treatment for a wound, as he felt others needed more help then he – a very brave thing to do, but it left my grandfather fatherless. No one would mess with Grandfather D. He was quite a character, and he lived life to the full. Like me, he had an eye for the girls. But he was also committed to his wife and his family. He taught us how to respect people and rules. His soul was so strong that his spirit added to all the other ones living in that very old beautiful country house. He and his wife were living in the small keeper's cottage attached to an old elegant haunted mansion. For a long time, we – me, my brother, sister and cousins – would feel his spirit and essence so much that it was scary and exciting at once.

My paternal grandmother lived till she was 92 years of age and was the only grandparent who saw my darkest manic side. As a very old lady, she freed her brain completely and would get quite high too. People call that dementia, but I would rather think that it is another step into freedom. Finally, at the end of their journey, people can let it go and allow themselves a complete and utter break from their heavy, educated principles.

One day just before the end, when I was in a kind of a manic state, she grabbed my hand in both of hers and said: 'I understand you Charlie, I know you're gonna make it!' She was the only person to be proud of my soft insanity.

Whether it is hard smoking, enjoying a drink or two or getting a natural high, it seems that my grandparents' bad habits dropped a generation and all landed on me, as much as their strong spirits and loving virtues and sins did. My lifestyle is a kind of homage to their existence, a concentration of fun and love; even though I look like a real alcoholic when I walk, and that is the strong impression I give people when they first see me. This is the reason why I need to tell them right away that I have MS, that I used to be a striker and am now bipolar.

The love of my grandparents has certainly supported me through the bad times; even if they weren't around, this paramount love has solidified me. Their spirit will nurture my very soul until the day I die. Thank you!

High-spirited and hazardous holidays

From European lineage, growing up in Africa and falling for each other in North America, my parents are citizens of the world and have the travelling bug. They worked very hard, not only to raise their children properly but also to allow the family brilliant and regular travel, especially as we had good friends and family all around the world. I knew I was a very lucky boy to be able to discover all these different cultures, climates, landscapes and, moreover, people. France, Turkey, Spain, Greece, Norway, Kenya, Sri Lanka, etc., anywhere I would find new friends even though I couldn't speak the language. It was natural for me to go and get involved in the gatherings of local children and their games. Whenever there was football and chess, I would join in and impress.

When I was seven, we went to visit my mother's cousin in Africa. Her husband was a cotton and coffee farmer and a safari guide and they lived in this lovely cottage on the tourist resort of Diani beach, where we stayed for a month at Christmas time. I discovered and fell in love with the tropics and its lifestyle. It was so different from anything I had ever seen. I was initiated to windsurf at seven years old, with my cousins' mates, and had a great experience on the board, carried on their shoulders. We had the best peaceful family holiday in the sun. I was like a little sponge, enjoying every minute of paradise life and witnessing the class- and race-divide of this world as something bizarre and normal at the same time.

When I was 13, we went to visit a good family friend in Asia. The first excitement on the way was a stopover in Dubai. The five-star hotel we stayed in was a palace of 1,001 nights, with grandiose architecture and decoration. It was even more exciting than being on a film set. We only had time to visit the jewel market. Even if I am losing my memory – especially when I'm tired – I can still visualise those treasures of gold and colourful beads. I was struck by the wealth of that growing country and the richness of its culture. It had nothing to do with the over-commercial, vulgar and fake resort that it quickly became. But I do understand how shiny, colourful, exotic wealth can be attractive and seductive.

On this holiday we stayed in a beautiful colonial house that appeared to me to be a mansion. I was discovering another aspect of colonial life, with servants at our disposal, playing croquet in the amazing tropical garden and drinking Pimms. Even more exciting were the local spiritual festivities. The most outstanding was this guy walking on hot coals in the woods. He was so focussed and blessed with holy spirits that he could do that without any pain. Above all, the most memorable encounters were with a local religious group who we thought were friendly local people but in fact were extremely dangerous terrorists. This group was fighting for their religious beliefs and rights and their revolutionary representatives were willing to create an independent state. We could feel the situation was very hot with local disruptions.

A visit to one of the hot spot areas was the place where I really sensed the tension. This beautiful Buddhist city in the north-east of the country has always also been a strategic political harbour. It was a city where, at the time, the fearless revolutionary soldiers of the opposition, the force behind the revolt, were hanging out. The ongoing tension was even more furious, as there was a presidential election campaign going on. We heard about this group killing people by cutting off their necks. The hotel was on a beach, which was where the revolutionary soldiers were also hanging out.

My older friends were very interested to find out what exactly was going on and directly went to talk to them and asked them all sorts of questions. The discussion went on for a such a long time that they even offered us drinks. When our parents found out who we hanging out with, they got really worried. It may have become a very dangerous situation for all of us. However, my friends were intelligent and genuine enough not to get into any stupid chat and tell them about their father's job (one that would have put us at risk). They knew who they were talking to but I just saw some nice blokes and was very shocked when I learnt they were dangerous people. That has been a great lesson to me not to always go by your first impressions and to understand that very nice people can be extremely dangerous. It seems that I can be attracted by that type of person and I may also be a kind of Dr Jekyll and Mr Hide myself.

Next stop was a magical town on the top of a hill surrounded by beautiful landscapes and inhabited by loads of holy spirits. Elephants seemed to be the holiest beings in this town, living in the temples, working and being fondly taken care of as well. I had seen elephants in Africa but never living among people and being so respected, especially during the religious festivities where they were treated as gods. We were so lucky to be there during the Elephant Festival. They were so beautiful, dressed up to the max with colourful or golden adornments and amazing make-up. I realised how powerful these animals are, able to be both dangerous and cool, potentially very submissive as well.

Then the ten of us drove to the centre of the island and went to stay on a tea plantation for a couple of days. One evening the whole family decided to play 'murder in the dark'. We set up a real drama in the house. Fun and fear was buzzing around. It worked dramatically, with screams and shouts, as we probably needed to release the tension gathered up by the beach. In the morning, we were shocked to hear that the villagers around the house thought that the rebels had killed us all.

The most horrific event in that red-hot journey was the true vision of a man burning alive in a tyre, as we were driving though the countryside in a rebel area. That is one of the worse things I have ever witnessed in my life. We were all horrified, couldn't express anything. I'd rather believe that he committed suicide but he may have been executed. My mother says that we never ever witnessed this but were told that it happened regularly and even that it was perpetuated by the government forces. This has shocked me so much that it has become a vivid memory in my brain. It seems to happen quite regularly to me that strong emotions create such intense memories or feelings that they become lucid in my mind.

After these emotional events and the whole country being closed down, we were quite happy to travel to a heavenly nearby archipelago. Because of rising political tension, our friend advised us to go to a tiny island where he knew nothing would happen. There, I discovered another paradise-on-earth or rather, under water. I was a good swimmer and loved snorkelling around, meeting with locals: turtles, thousands of different colourful shiny fish, dancing plants. That was heaven. I found a new interest in shells, such diverse and beautiful shapes and colours. Crustaceans have such beautiful homes! I can also remember a boat trip surrounded by a reef of little sharks. I was tempted to jump in and swim with them.

Even though I am losing my memory, long- and short-term, and especially that photographic memory I had been so proud of, that trip to Asia holds the strongest images of my beautiful childhood holidays. At 13 years old I was understanding how mystical and confusing this world can be, with heaven and hell living together as one in the name of God. I had always been interested in those mysteries of life.

As you will learn in reading about my Jesus Christ saga, religion has always been a part of my existence, and especially part of my unconscious. I am a believer; even if I don't clearly know who is my God, I do believe in higher powers. Even if it is a bit out of context in this holiday chapter, I am happy to remember what an excellent student I was in Religious Education. I enjoyed it very much for several reasons: the teacher was stunningly beautiful and I was almost in love with her. She appreciated my artwork so much that my arts skills improved a lot during those studies. I was also drawn to that subject because of my mum. Even though she never talked about religion at all, I felt it was in her and I was inspired by the fact that she had been to convent school. I knew that her spiritual beliefs are the source of her amazing natural loving power and undeniable strength in life. Actually, I could even feel her presence in RE class. There is certainly some sort of Oedipus complex there, projecting the huge love for my mum to the teacher in a holy way to make it more acceptable.

Brecon Beacons in Wales was the favourite magical holiday spot where we escaped to as often as possible. We rented a derelict little cottage for peanuts opposite my father's good friend from university. He worked in London too but preferred to live in the countryside and commuted every day. His wife got along really well with Mum, and their three children were all similar ages to us. Their house was the coolest because they had a bar downstairs and lots of fun was had there.

Life in Wales was so brilliantly different from London life. Breathtaking landscapes made me feel as small as a mouse and as large as a giant. Waking up every morning in that valley was like enjoying a fairy tale, especially as we were completely free. Our friends' youngest child was my best friend and showed me all kind of local excitements; hiking, fishing, barbecuing, swimming, hunting, etc. He was a great fisherman and was very good at clay pigeon shooting as well. Now he fishes for money and jumps from one company to another, always true to himself and his values. Although he was a bit younger than me, he reached puberty before me. He told me all kind of stories about his girlfriends and what they would get up to out in the wild. It seemed that nature was inviting them to take part and open up their instincts. It sounded far more exciting and genuine than those porn movies I came across with mates in their London pads. I was very intrigued with these stories but definitely not ready for that kind of action yet. Football and nature were more appealing to me than the female form. In the middle of those mountains and valleys, waterfalls, various lights and many surprising sights full of animal life, each moment was a blessing. Wales was my peaceful place.

When MS and bipolar started and I couldn't in anyway dare think of flying away with my friends to shag the world, Wales was still the best place to rest and feel blessed with life, forgetting about illness and feeling in harmony with the universe. With hindsight, I believe I was developing a wild animal nature which is the favourite and usual side of my bipolarity.

My stupendous parents

My parents are just incredible and amazing. Both my parents were born in East Africa. It is very fortunate that they met in a Polish delicatessen in Quebec and connected right away with their East African twang. They are such a great match and have so much respect for each other; they are always each other's ally and know they have each other's back. Anyone can sense their love for one another even though they don't kiss and touch each other in front of us. When they have an argument, Dad just walks away and Mum can go into a powerful silence state, preferably in the garden or with a book, her places of solace. That taught me how to respect people's emotions in leaving them alone to process their negative feelings, inside and out. It was a very useful technique to get my girlfriends back after a dispute. I am hoping to find the love of my life like my parents have.

I feel blessed by both my parents – THANK YOU. I am the luckiest man in the world, even though their house can be my place of solace and a prison hell at the same time. To many people such a paradox may sound bizarre, but that is my reality.

My father is an honourable and admirable man. He has never told a real lie in his life, which I wish was the same for me. He is soft, sweet and generous, plus very intelligent. He knows how to be strict without being rough. Something that impressed me a lot about him was that he listened to classical music when he was revising for university. He is a very calm man who rarely shouts, only when I really drive him crazy. I am very fortunate and proud to have a father like him who is loved by all. I know how much Dad loves me. He is the one who encouraged my football passion in taking me to Tottenham Hotspur home games as a young boy, and then he would try not to miss any of my games. He was my first fan whilst I was playing and would always celebrate my skills. But at home he would still be very attentive to my school results and my behaviour. If I was naughty, he would flick me on the back of the head, which would wake me up instantly. I really appreciate the way I was brought up. When both my parents were unhappy about me, they would tell me, once, clearly and would just leave it there without further discussion or negative attitude.

My dad loves his cricket and I have seen cricket matches with him so many times. All generations and all social classes would meet at these games and the atmosphere was electric. Dad was also, and still is, a golf player. Unfortunately, he has now got the degenerative illness Parkinsons and he is losing his strength and his 'oomph', except when Mum is around. He is still so much in love with her: her presence makes him feel secure and happy. As a matter of fact, Mum is the pillar of security within this family.

Without the guidance and dedication of my mum, I would be six feet under. I have always trusted her the most. Even in the middle of a big argument, I know I can trust her, which makes me even more frustrated; I can never win with her. We tend to connect in a very good way. She is such a powerful woman. She trained as a nurse at a London hospital where the royal family gives birth. Then she went to work for three years in Canada where she first met Dad. She then decided to travel around South America for ten months with two girlfriends. That was during the Vietnam War and they met a lot of draft dodgers who were doing amazing work in various poor communities of South America. They got involved with a local development doctor and nursed at his clinic.

This trip convinced her to get more involved in development organisations; she worked with War on Want and then decided to train in London as a health visitor and later as a family planning nurse. She got married and started working in some of the poorest areas of London. While Dad was working in the city, Mum was in the rougher sides of town. One day when she was seven months pregnant with my good self, she got threatened with a fake gun by a father. With her wise and gentle ways, she managed to get out with her heart pounding. I believe I did an overhead kick in her womb but I am sure that this event made me feel even more secure in her womb rather than anxious. Mum realised she was putting her family at risk and decided to stop working in this area and with community work, especially when I came along. My arrival may have kick-started her creative side, as she then joined a stained-glass course. Mum always liked to draw sketches. I was especially impressed and inspired by those from her South American trip. She has always been extremely interested in all kind of arts. She opened her young children's minds to the arty side of life and instilled us with a love for beauty and that creative energy that opens us up to our own souls.

My mother is a powerhouse and my love for her reaches beyond everything. In existence on this planet and beyond, I know our souls will be together forever as they are now, even when she makes me feel furious. Eternal love does not exclude exasperation at times. She is a radiant lady with so much to give. She stuck by me through thick and thin throughout my illnesses, always making my ladies a cup of tea in the morning, making sure I keep on the straight and narrow, which I often stray from. She is the busiest lady I have ever came across and at the same time she always manages to be available. Everyone who meets her enjoys her input into everything.

The true beauty of my mum's attributes are far and wide. She is a wise old owl. By the way, she knows these birds quite well. She always has a natural helping hand for any living being. When she was a young child in Malaysia, she saved dogs from monsoon drains. Later, near Lake Victoria in Tanzania, she persuaded her parents to buy a little otter that was tied up in a tiny cage. She called her Otterlina and managed to find a fisherman who trained the otter to seek out fish in the lake so that she could be freed into the water. Because she travelled a lot as a child, she was used to leaving friends and loved ones behind and had to build new relationships in every new home. This is certainly how she developed this special sensitivity to social inclusion.

She was a kind of hippy when she was young but never did any drugs. Her radiant character can lighten up a whole party. She seems to enjoy taking care of every single individual's need as much as enjoying partying. Her internal strength is such that anyone can feel the effects of her shining soul. When she is tired and upset, it will also affect the mood of the whole house.

The garden is her place of solace. She can stop caring for everyone's needs when she decides to buy flowers or work in the garden, but she would always kindly let people know it's garden time, which means her own 'me time' to recharge her batteries and gather her thoughts. She has quite a few other personal activities such as yoga, film and book groups. Moreover, she enjoys her weekly day off to visit her grandchildren.

She can also take a little break to go and read in the park or meet friends. She is a book lover and has got an impressive collection. Of course, she has read everything about learning disabilities, MS and Parkinson's; she has read so much about bipolar syndrome and manic behaviour, trying to understand and help me. How strange and serendipitous! Those plentiful hardcore challenges have fallen upon the shoulders of the only person on earth able to deal with such heavy load. Is it bad luck or a blessing? It seems that our close family has concentrated the whole extended clan's history of neurologic, mental and genetic illnesses. We manage to make the juice of this concentrate quite sweet though, as we all have a huge sense of love, positivity and humour. Even more, I also tend to make it glamorous so I can swallow it more pleasurably, relying on my family to keep me in touch with reality.

However, Mum knows that she needs support as well. Twenty-three years ago with a bunch of good friends, Mum set up a fantastic organisation in the field of disability. This experience has been invaluable for her to get through all the administration bollocks and find the support we both need. It must have helped her a lot to share her burden, but it must also have taken so much energy. By the way, she *hates* the word burden. If she thought it was a burden, she would feel like a victim in some trap, but she does not and that is how she can happily cope with the situations. And it is also how she taught me to be so positive. A few years ago, as my dad was diagnosed with Parkinson, she stopped working for this charity. They miss her a lot, and I feel that she would still benefit from that sharing and support – especially now that she is reaching her seventies and still has three disabled men's lives to organise. This demands the powers of an angel.

She has always had a dream to go to India and with the income from this book I hope that I can send her there. In the meantime, once every few years, she manages to go away somewhere in Europe for a week or two. To make sure we are safe at home in her absence, she organises everything to a T with a bunch of friends and family with all the trimmings paid for. It is difficult for me to cope without her constant love and care. We all miss her heavily, it hurts, but then we must let it go and explore our own island without motherhood.

For instance, I take advantage of her not being around to do silly things that make everyone furious: I stole and drank my dad's gin and tonic plus his glass of wine when he was away to the toilet, and Matt the spy told him. I know it was stupid, I felt silly but Dad and I were in the same boat, drinking to forget Mum's absence. Matt is also drinking a bit more than usual but I can see that he is controlling the situation better than Dad and myself. I don't mind Matt spying on me because I am used to his amazing honesty (this honesty split me up from many girlfriends) and I know it is good for me to have this honest man on my side. His emotional intelligence is massive, he instinctively knows how to control his negative feelings and not get overwhelmed by them. When Mum is away, I am even more aware of the huge work she does to organise our wellbeing and of her unconditional loving care. Now I also realise it is good to talk about it and let the pain of her absence out. This book is very helpful to become mindful of my emotions, to accept them and move on, because it's time to groove on. I love you Mum, you're amazing.

Although I have been very nice about my mother, I must say that she can be witchlike when she is over-controlling me. Unfortunately, she has got no choice but to manage a house full of vulnerable people, including a young adult with MS and bipolar. She is a fantastic matriarch. It is tricky for me to feel so dependent on my mum or sometimes on my sister. It makes me feel even more vulnerable, as I cannot give back, cannot protect and support them. That huge frustration in the face of the most respected and loved women in my life can make me a bit aggressive with them sometimes. Fortunately, they know how to stop me right away by showing me that being offensive is not my real self, so I don't feel guilty for too long.

Layla, a stronghold beauty

Sometimes when a family battle is getting hot, my sister Layla intervenes as a mediator, even though she lives about an hour away. She will call me and try to turn down the heat by explaining my parents' arguments and defending them while understanding my situation as well. She is just two years older than me and has always been my protector, a role model and my best friend as well. We went to the same school, supporting each other and sharing loads of games, especially during holidays. She can be quite emotional and solid at the same time. My trial has been a real challenge for her as well, and still is. When I was stuck in hospital, she would send me lovely tender poems or deep letters. Their poignancy would lift me up with their unconditional love and understanding. A few years ago, I got a place at a specialist unit and this is the letter she sent:

> Darling Bro – I just wanted to say how incredibly proud we all are of you and your attitude about taking this opportunity on. You really do deserve to focus on you and your understanding what inner strength you have and have always had inside in order to make you strong and to live life in a way that is rewarding, independent but also safe away from the 'wolves'!!
>
> You are such an amazing brother, full of love energy and laughter and at important times have an incredible wisdom. You also very importantly are the BEST UNCLE in the world – along with our lovely brother Matt – who also loves you very much.
>
> Mum and Dad are very proud of you and all they want is for you to be happy and centred. They love you more than the moon the sun and the world. You are very cherished – don't ever forget that.
>
> Here is a circle-of-life pendant to remind you that we all love you. Lots of love, Layla

She went to an art college and then university, where she did performing arts. She performed with a theatre company before she met her husband and made two amazing lovely children, my niece and nephew. They live just outside of London where their enchanting house and garden are a safety net for the whole family. Layla and her husband regularly welcome Matt and I for a weekend when our parents are going for a much-needed break. She can be very tough sometimes in a motherly manner, especially when I smoke in the house. Unfortunately, I love to break the rules, and it is easier for me to do so at my sister's than at my parents' house – not fair for Layla and her young family. Layla also wants family time when we go out together and I talk to every individual who I come across in the street. Everyone in my entourage gets annoyed about it too.

My niece and nephew are certainly the most lovable people in my world, and they love me. I am a good uncle: playing, teaching, hugging. One of my favourite games is Catch – I can't kick, but I *can* catch! Whatever they're playing, I'll participate and I enjoy them engaging so easily with my free spirit. I also dig being the teacher and showing them good manners, even though it may be difficult for me to have good manners. I also realise that I sometimes enjoy being the controlling adult with them. Of course, they are the only human beings I can have a bit of power over. No worries – I never overuse that power. Individual dignity is too important!

At the end of 2014, we learnt the horrific news that Layla had been diagnosed with the same illness as me, even though MS is never the same. It hurts so deeply that I still have difficulties talking about it; plus, I feel this is too private for me to comment on. I will just admit that this news had such an impact on my neurologic system that my bladder system went spare and buggered up on me. I am very pissed off to know that she is in the same rocking boat as me; it hurts a lot, so much that we cannot even talk about it together.

Here is Layla's letter to me written after we finished the book and before she had yet read it. She was very concerned that her frankness would hurt me. It was very emotional and sad indeed to be reminded what she has been, and still is, going through because of me, what an impact it has on her life. However, I did know all that. I can only say how sorry and mournful I am.

> 8 November 2017
>
> To my very special brother,
>
> Firstly I want to say how very proud I am of you and Mab for creating this book together. It is an incredible achievement and a testi-

mony to both your determination to never give up and your enormous respect for one another. This process has enabled you to share your thoughts and reveal your stories and I hope this will become a document from which many people learn more about what it might look and feel like in your world. I also hope that the contributions from professionals who have worked with you and the many family and friends who love you will enrich and contextualise some of your stories and give further insight into your amazing, valued and important life.

Love and labels

I love you so very deeply my darling brother. I am your older sister by two years and we share our wonderful younger brother Matt who is five years younger than me and three years younger than you. We are lucky enough to have had an adventurous, wonderful, loving and supportive mum and dad who have managed, sometimes against serious odds, to nourish and continue to develop a very loving extraordinary family. Matt was born with a learning disability and I feel that sharing a brother as special and as loving as Matt, brought us, at an early age, very close together. We formed a strong bond between us that was about celebrating Matt as our brother, loving him for him and loving us for us. We had the freedom of not understanding what the 'syndrome' Matt was labelled with meant. We had no idea of what ramification society's fear of 'difference' might potentially hold for Matt's future. We were free of that baggage and could love him for who he was and celebrate him as our younger sibling. We had the freedom of not knowing that in the future at different times both of us would become ill.

Happy days

For many years this was a time of freedom and childhood innocence. Whilst I remember fierce hair-pulling battles and arguments about who sat where in the car, my abiding memories from that time are of real happiness. Long, wet, windy holidays in a 'Withnail and I' cottage in Wales. Fishing, BBQs and endless days of swimming by the river with very best friends. Wonderful walks, real fires, hot chocolate and playing endless games as a family. Weekends spent with lovely grandparents, aunties, uncles and cousins in their beautiful gardens, big get-togethers with love and laughter, tree-climbing, swimming in lakes and adventuring. Amazing holidays to faraway places with family and friends. You, brave and strong and so young on the shoulders of a wind surfer, us spending all day snorkelling, jumping into wild waves and swimming with basking sharks. Waiting up most of the night to catch Father Christmas and the excitement of bulging stockings full of presents on Christmas morning. I can see your beautiful face and excited expression – so full of life and exuberance. I remember days where many children would tumble back to our house in London, hot crumpets and butter, sugar donuts and jam, creating plays, hide-and-seek, sardines, fireworks parties, birthday parties and trips to the cinema and theatre. Sunday night 'A-Team' and scrambled eggs, cherished pets that came and went. I remember too your love and extraordinary talent for football, the skill you had on the field and the immense feeling of pride we all had for you. I don't ever remember you being arrogant about this, you just lived the game and the game loved you living it. I remember you never having to study, but always got everything right and I also remember most of my friends falling for your beautiful charm and cheeky wit. Happy happy days.

Celebration of difference

Of course, alongside all of this as Matt got older we noticed people staring and sometimes got a sense of people's embarrassment, of not knowing quite where to look or what to say. I know that you, at times had to endure some cruel bullying about Matt at primary school, an experience I was lucky enough never to have had to confront. As a sister, I always felt so very proud of Matt, so ready to take the world on and to stare back at those who stared – wanting them to know – actually how lucky we were to have Matt in our family. When people asked about my brothers, they would often say they were 'sorry' when I told them that Matt had a learning disability. My response to this was to tell them why I wasn't 'sorry' and why he was so important to us and in fact how lucky we were. I know how hurtful that bullying must have been and I know you love Matt as much as I do. It somehow feels important to highlight these beginnings of our life together as siblings. A fierce sense of protection and a celebration of 'difference'.

Trauma of the unknown

I want to try and explain the reality of, as Mum would say, 'walking the walk' alongside you, my deeply loved brother who has now been ill for nearly 25 years of my 43-year life. Whose illness is so complex and indeed changeable that it has at times been impossible to tell people 'what' it is that you have, to tell people why it is you sometimes behave in the way you do and to explain why I wouldn't change who you are for the world. In a way the beginning of this experience was the polar opposite of my experience of Matt, people would often not know what multiple sclerosis was or indeed bipolar – many of your symptoms were invisible and can be interpreted in the wrong way. So if you stumble, people think you're on drugs, if you slur, people think you're drunk, if you say something inappropriate, people think you are just rude. Matt was automatically 'given' a medical label – this happened as soon he was born. A label which is weighed down heavy with certain assumptions made as soon as someone looks at his beautiful face. Things were very different when you first became ill. Of course, Matt is not ill; his learning disability is not an illness. People like Matt are dis-abled because of societies' responses to them. When you became ill there was no clear 'label' which people could cling to, no clear course of treatment to 'cure' you, everything was colliding, not clear-cut – there was no way of knowing how to support you and your rights to be free. There was no way of knowing how to sometimes literally keep you alive. You were certainly dis-abled by your illness and societies response to you having it. My experience of having a new 'dis-abled' brother was very different to the known experience I had been used to. I think it's important to think about what has 'dis-abled' you. However, I also think it's as important to think about what factors have also allowed you to be free. By this I mean being free in ways that so many people crave and strive to be in their lives. You, my wild wonderful brother, have been able to throw off the shackles of inhibition. In fact, many of us would love to shed those shackles in the 'we only live once' lives we lead. We are too restrained and scared to be different and free in our actions and thoughts, to take risks like you have, to run to the unknown and embrace it for everything it has to offer.

Telling the 'story'

When you first became ill, we, as a family had to learn very quickly new ways of talking about you, new ways of telling our close family and friends about your illness and new ways of dealing with society's fear of difference. Indeed, we had to face full frontal our own fears of what was happening. We also realised that not everyone could deal with what was going on, even people who loved you. This is a complex and scary time when you learn so much about people you thought you knew, mostly good things but sometimes painful things, sometimes you feel let down by them and feel thoroughly alone. As a sister I had to learn a new way of protecting you as my little brother, I also had to learn how to protect (in my way) Matt and my mum and dad. No one ever told me I had to do this, it is just what I needed to do as a big sister. I remember your diagnosis of MS and bipolar as a deeply shocking period of my life. I have only recently realised that it was and indeed sometimes continues to be an experience of Trauma. We were all trying to look after you and somehow within that to also look after ourselves and each other. We were trying to manage the distress, fear and frustration of other people who loved you and were also confused and frightened by your diagnosis. There were no guide-books on this, we were literally making it up as we went along. This is especially true in the early days of your extreme behaviour.

Low times

The years have meshed into each other, I guess it's not that important *when* things happened but that they are significant, because I remember them. In one of your very low periods I remember walking into my bedroom in which I thought you were sleeping to see you trying to climb out of the window very distressed – to this day I don't know if you were trying to kill yourself or if it were a cry for help. I remember running to 'catch' you and then not wanting to leave you. I nearly left university because it felt too far for me to get to you and make you safe. I remember your extreme highs, with you walking out on the street with no clothes on, blessing passers-by, because you literally thought you were Jesus Christ incarnated. I remember you breaking the glass on Mum's beautiful stained-glass door because they were trying to keep you safe by keeping you in. You were never violent towards us but had a new-found strength and power which you were determined to use to get out of the house. I remember sitting with you deep into the night, you refusing your medication and you playing songs to me over and over again for hours. You were trying to make me understand what you were trying to say through the music playing as if the words of the songs were yours and yours alone – I remember not knowing how to make you stop. It felt like raw and emotional torture. I remember not being able to stop physically shaking when I went out with you to a bar because I never knew what you would say or do next. I remember many people finding you so attractive, interesting and wild – you were the buzz of the party, the centre of everything – you would always be drawn to the person who could match your energy and risk-taking. I remember never being able to let go, never being able to relax, always fearful that your mouth, your body, your mind would lead you to danger. This sounds extreme but the fact is that my fears would often come to fruition. I remember some acute periods of anxiety in the early days. Some that are seared on my memory are when you were 'voluntarily' sectioned and then beaten up by the staff, all the times you went missing and were located in the early hours in some really dangerous area, when I found out you had been smoking crack, when I found out that dealers were coming into our house. I mostly feel sad about when I knew you were lying to me, our friends and mum and dad, and as much as I understood on so many levels why you would lie it, felt so deeply sad and at that time really affected how much I could take. There were times when I had to walk away.

Wild ways

But, who could blame you for your wild ways, I somehow feel that when you have been manic, your mind has somehow protected you from the reality of MS. A disease with unpredictable and unknown future. Your consultants couldn't tell us what, when and how your MS would next manifest. Even when your challenges have been so huge – you would often say you were happy and that you loved your life – you would embrace each day as if it were a new adventure, you would constantly ask me if I was happy and tell me that you loved me. You never complained, you never got bitter, you never seemed jealous – you loved deeply, took and accepted people at face value. You were so often charming and clever and funny. You had (and still have in a way) many things going on and many 'labels' converging. What you have had to deal with in your life is deeply complex and not simple to treat, to put into words, to understand. Multiple sclerosis, which has changed from an original diagnosis of relapsing remitting MS (to now a diagnosis of progressive MS) is a disease that affects everyone differently. It is one that people still find very difficult to understand. Your diagnosis was at a time when medication was still in its infancy and your youth meant you were advised against drug therapy. Your MS symptoms have gone from not been able to stop being sick, to not being able to walk, to double incontinence, not being able to have sex, experiencing deep fatigue, not being able to swallow and in more recent years a devastating development of severe memory loss (and so many other things in-between). You also have brain damage to your frontal lobe from a very early 'MS attack' when you were very young and have also been diagnosed with bipolar disorder related to MS. This happened at a time when many people had no idea about what bipolar was. Bipolar and frontal lobe damage has meant you have had, in the past, a huge sex drive, an extraordinary imagination that has often crossed into fantasy, no inhibitions, no sense of danger to yourself and others, a degree of self-obsession and a constant need to push the boundaries and explore new and exciting things. In fact, as a child of the 'rave' generation, it often felt like you acted as though you were constantly on ecstasy (even when you weren't!). You would cross a busy road with no fear of being hit and no understanding of the dangers of that hazardous behaviour for you or indeed others – and that kind of sums up how you lived your life. You had a feeling of freedom, release and excitement that many of our friends were enthralled by when first discovering ecstasy. The chemical imbalance in your brain meant you were at times on a huge rush and limitless high.

When illness strikes

Whilst you have a small group of defiantly loyal and wonderful friends, many of the core group of school friends quickly disappeared from your life. They couldn't cope with you as a friend, it was far too much of a challenge and they didn't have the maturity to be able to stick with you. There is no blame associated with this, just the very sad reality of what happens when illness both mental and physical strikes someone down at such a formative and vulnerable age. It's a double blow where you lose so much control over your body and mind and you also then lose many of the people around you to keep you steady and safe. As a sister, there was no way that I was going to abandon you – our life together has been an 'interesting' ride, my darling brother.

Words and actions

You may notice that the words 'interesting', 'walk the walk' and 'journey' come up a few times. These words are ones that have been constantly repeated in our family and reflect an approach of how we have tried to support you in the highs and the lows. These words, plus a whole barrel full of love and deep respect for you, have held us all together and allowed us all to survive.

Positivity and guilt

I have to admit that sometimes this 'journey' with you has been full of pain. I cannot deny that there has at times been a deep pool of sadness that has bubbled beneath the happy exterior we as a family give off. Much of the time we have been fire-fighting for your survival and at the core we have never given up on you. I want to make it very clear that the trauma is there only because we are so full of love and respect for you. As you know, we have also been led by who you call fondly your 'matriarch' mother, your ally, your friend, your political activist, your defender and your rock. Our amazing mum, whose positive vision meant that at times we actually didn't have a choice but to carry on, that we had to get through certain times because to pause and reflect may have led to collapse. Dad, has at times been more expressive about his deep pain about your illness and its repercussions – you know that he loves you so very much and is very proud of you. He has supported Mum every step of the way. I wonder if Mum's positivity is also her 'coping' mechanism, if she didn't have this amazing ability I'm not sure she could have achieved all she has for you and us as a family. I remember when I first became a mum realising just how much she has loved us and just how much pain she at times must have been through. Matt is always there for you, as your partner in crime, your brother and your beer buddy and latterly someone who always makes sure you're alright and that you have everything you need. We have somehow managed to bring all our different opinions, thoughts, fears and love to the pot and have somehow kept this family strong. I'm sure you would agree that without your family around you – advocating and fighting for your right to be heard, your right to be informed about and involved in making decisions about your treatment – life would have been very different. As Mum says, there is dignity in risk. People who have survived traumatic times love deep and strong and as your sister, as well as experiencing pain, my time with you has often felt like a gift.

The illness and not you

It would be ridiculous to pretend that at times I don't still go to a dark place. Your illness has had repercussions for everyone around you.

It took me a long time to accept that it was the illness and not you that was at times steering you on a scary and worrying course. This was particularly true with some of your behaviour associated with bipolar and frontal lobe damage. Your illness and the isolation it has created around you has made you attracted to vulnerable people and vice versa and it has without doubt led you to do dangerous things. But I can totally understand the seduction of always wanting to live your life to the full and on the edge, to up the high through drugs, to up the high through danger or sensual pleasure. It has been especially hard to 'walk the walk' when the physical and mental come-downs from 'binging' on danger have been so destructive to your health and well-being. I wonder if I will ever be brave enough to tell you that I have sometimes mourned a brother that could have been, imagined a brother without illness, that sometimes I have felt deep sadness at losing (through your illness) a different kind of sibling best friend, a confidant that I have never been able to have. That sometimes it has been hard to not see Mum and Dad as much because they need to be there for you and Matt. How can I say that without feeling excruciating guilt at even thinking that – these are thoughts that feel at times like raw cuts on the surface and at other times are deeply buried for my own self-protection and the protection of others.

When words don't work

Five years ago, I was also diagnosed with MS. This brought up so many feelings and fears relating to my future and the 'path' this illness would take me on. It also gave me some deeper insight and huge admiration for you and how you have confronted this devastating illness. I knew that without therapy of some sort I didn't feel that I would survive even the diagnosis stage. During therapy I was shocked at the amount of time I needed to talk through the real pain that I felt about you being ill, the repercussions for our family and my responses to it. At times the sadness was so deep that I couldn't even find any words – the fear, particularly of you dying, left me mute and in indescribable pain.

Wouldn't change you for the world

I have thought for many months about how I can navigate this look back on our 'journey' as brother and sister in a way that doesn't somehow let you down, reveal too much about your life, reveal too much about myself, reveal mistakes, reveal pain. I chose to write my words without having read your words first, I didn't want what you had written to influence my contribution, I wonder how much our memories and thoughts will connect. Most of all, I want to make sure that people know why I wouldn't change you for the world and that not everything has been sad. In fact there have been such happy and special times, such hysterical and bizarre moments, such deep love between us all that I often feel lucky. Lucky to have loved and thought about love, to have been able to say the things that pressurised situations make you say, to not be inhibited by the normal social norms. I want to celebrate the very happy, rich and fulfilling life we have had as a family and how vital and central you have been to that happiness and celebration. I want to acknowledge the extraordinary support group of people who love you and our family very deeply and have been there for us in the most wonderful of ways. I want to highlight some unique professionals who have gone that extra step to see you as a human being in all that complexity and not just a client who exists in a clinic. Your eccentric ways, as well as at times putting you and us in danger, have also made us laugh so loudly, as well as cry so hard. How you have attracted unique and interesting people to you and our family. How our life has been richer by knowing some of your friends, the carers who are with you many times a day and your amazing personal assistants. Many of these people have become central not just to you but to our family as a whole. My children adore you, their very special uncle Charlie, you may not play the same way other uncles play, or indeed say what other uncles say – but how you play and what you say is just as important to them. There was a moment a few years ago at my house, before you had to use a wheelchair, when you could just about still make it up the stairs and we ran you a lovely relaxing bath. I was on my own and I struggled to get you out of the bath and up onto the bed to get your dressed. As you lay naked on the floor of the upstairs hall you looked at me straight in the eye and said 'Did you ever imagine our life would be like this'. You said it with such grace and sensitivity, such humanity and gentleness. I replied that I never imagined that our life would be like this but that I loved you very much. Living this life with you is part of why I am who I am, why I think the way I think, why I have the strong relationship I have and why I am lucky enough to have deep friendships. It is also part of the reason why my young children love as deep as they do and are as perceptive and wise as they sometimes are. There are many things to be positive about. You, my darling brother, are one of them. You will

> always be in our hearts wherever we may journey. Thanks for walking the walk with me my darling bro, it's been so much more than interesting.
> I love you to the moon and back.
> Love Layla

Clan members

Everyone knows that family is crucial in life. But in my own circumstances it has been simply vital, because of the way my illness has changed my life and their lives too. It is clear that it was very difficult to understand my condition for some time. My behaviour must be very annoying, especially when I lick plates or when I keep on rapping or touching people, which is totally understandable. It is very painful at times, as I adore everybody around me. As a matter of fact, it took a while to get an official report explaining that my strange behaviour was a neurological problem and not my nature. With this understanding, people began to understand me and my behaviour more.

My family brought me love and respect and was there all the way through. I remember when my aunty, Dad's sister, cried during a hospital visit and I cried with her; that was one of the rare occasions when tears sprouted from my eyes. I felt so at home and balanced with her, it was good to be able to feel vulnerable, comfortable and secure at once, to feel the pain and be loved and understood, to be myself. She has a brilliant family and I remember many happy times with them. Same thing with my aunty Jeanne, the French lady who married my mum's brother David. I have always got along so well with her. She would do anything for me, as if I was her own son. She is always so generous towards me, with her time and warm energy, in the less appealing situations when I need personal care. Because she doesn't live with me all the time, she is amazingly patient and sweet with me. She is also a real talent in the kitchen, cooking the best dishes, while her incredible laugh intoxicates me. I feel blessed to have her as an aunty in my life. Her husband David is my mum's brother. They make such an amazing couple, often having Matt and I for weekends to allow my parents to have a break. This was always a lot of fun for both of us. Here is what she says about me:

> I first met you in 1993, when your uncle David introduced me to the family. I so remember our first meeting: you were going to France with your school and you asked me how you could chat up the French girls! I came up with a few boring words and eventually a crucial line:

'Ne t'inquiète pas …' (the rest of the sentence is between the two of us!). We often talk about this but I have never asked you if you have actually used it? Anyway, I am always so impressed that you still remember it and pronounce it so well.

I have very fond memories of you at our wedding in Devon (especially you chasing our young friends Lilly, Katy and Annabel …) and during the French marriage playing cricket in the field in front of the Chateau. Happy times!

So many other happy family occasions when, even with your difficulties, you are the star of the show. It is wonderful to see you surrounded by your friends and family.

You are an amazing artist and I am so privileged to have some of your art that you have generously given us over the years. I am now looking forward to reading your book.

You becoming ill has had a real affect in my life. I don't think I have ever met such an incredibly brave young man. You never complain and seem to always be in good spirit.

Your kind words towards me are very touching and I want you to know that I am here for you (even if I haven't been much around recently, sorry). You always make me feel so good and welcome, although I feel very sad when I think of your situation.

I love you very very much and you will always be in my heart.

Jeanne

My uncle, my mother's brother, has always been welcoming to me and I have had happy times with his family. He used to be a ladies' man, with a great style to pull the ladies, just like me. Before he got married, he would always bring home some really nice ladies. Maybe I got this individual and social ability from him. I always have adored my uncle, and still do. He is always coming up with unusual ideas for outdoor activities and family gatherings, like rounders on Boxing Day. We have had a lot of amazing times with his family. He has been very helpful to Mum over setting up spreadsheets to organise my support.

David's first wife was really beautiful and they have a son, Ralph, who is 15 years younger than me. He is such an amazing young man, very bright at school, and – just like me! – incredibly intelligent and beautiful. Because of the age difference, we didn't share many games or activities. I had already been diagnosed with MS when we managed to become closer. I would enjoy chatting with him at family gatherings and share with him my love stories. It may have helped him to understand about love and sex. He wouldn't mind telling me off sometimes. I wouldn't care much, as he is my cousin. I really enjoyed spending more time with him when he was my personal assistant (PA) during one summer. It was lovely to get closer to him. I love the way he talks about life. I feel that he has became both my brother and my best friend. See below an excerpt from Ralph about me:

> My experience with Charlie.
>
> My relationship with Charlie has always been a good one. I was the youngest child in the family. My cousins Layla, Charlie and Matt are all at least eight years older than me, so Charlie's quirks and idiosyncrasies were always a normal part of family life. I just accepted that Charlie was the way he was, being only five or six at the time that he was diagnosed. I think it is for this reason he doesn't exasperate me with his bullshit as much as he does other people.
>
> I am just old enough to remember watching Charlie playing football once before the MS, and I still remember how impressive he was with the ball and how rapidly he could suddenly take off down the field. Since then, I have seen Charlie go from being able to walk unaided, to using a stick, to being in a wheelchair. But again, thinking back on watching this process, it is very difficult to separate it from what would be considered 'normal' by other children. For me, what could be deemed an extraordinary situation was translated into a picture of an ordinary and loving family, which was made to seem effortless by the people around Charlie, mostly his mother – my aunt – Hannah, whom I know Charlie loves and respects more than anything, no matter how much he moans about her.
>
> When I was a child, Charlie used to take care of me when my parents went out for an evening. We would have a good time, playing board games, watching TV, ordering pizza. To this day, he still beats me at chess in an embarrassingly low number of moves.
>
> Later in life, when I was an adolescent and Charlie was in his twenties, I found it more and more difficult to get to know him and I started to understand why strangers didn't hang around long when they met. He tended to use the shock factor much more than he does now, making obscene jokes or coming on way too strong with any passing woman. It either made people laugh or feel uncomfortable – and nothing in-between. He still retains that ability but the wheelchair gives him a vulnerability that means people feel less threatened than they did when he could stand his full six-foot-one height.
>
> During my teenage years, I was more removed from the Bacchus household, having gone to boarding school, so even though we were

cousins, I really only saw Charlie at Christmas and at family gatherings. It is only in the past year that I have spent the most amount of time with him. I, like many others, spent the summer as his PA, playing chess together, going to the shops, to cycling sessions at the velodrome, to the gym and the cinema to watch whatever might be on. We had more conversations in these few months than in all the years before and it was then that I saw the amount of love and empathy that burns in Charlie. I could see that his family is the most important thing in the world to him. It still takes time for me to sift out all his bullshit but in-between all the stories of sleeping with 40,000 women and the dreams of becoming a millionaire, the wonderful things he says about those closest to him show me the respect and interest he holds for others.

My summer with Charlie has also made me see the best in people – or at least in the people in his community. Charlie will bring anyone into his conversation, no matter how far away they may be walking or how busy they might project themselves to seem, and to see people interact with him so politely and willingly has given me a confidence in humanity that I may have never really seen if I hadn't spent that summer with cousin Charlie.

Ralph

I know that I can be really annoying, especially to the people who are with me 24/7. At least they know why I'm like that and we always forgive each other. I know it is not the case in every family. This is why I feel so lucky with the family I have!

It is also very safe for me to know that my uncles and aunties would be 100 per cent behind my parents in any situation. I have such a magical family!

Crucial connections

My parents have this ability to make such good friends that we consider them as part of the family: going on holidays together, having parties as well as serious talks, supporting each other. It is good to know I have this other circle of people in my life, not too close, but loving enough to be able to rely on each other.

One very close lady in my life is my mother's great friend Cleo. She was married with my parents' great friend Geoff. I consider Cleo as my second mother, as I know she would always be there for me, with her beautiful smile and very bubbly personality. It is difficult to explain with words the special bond I feel for her. The speech she gave for my twenty-first birthday expresses it really well.

> Charlie was born beautiful and talented – and he has arrived at this milestone as beautiful and talented as ever. This is however not solely due to his birthright but also to a tremendous strength and ability to overcome adversity. My admiration knows no bounds. Geoff would by now be raving about his sporting prowess – not only his great gift as a footballer but latterly as an unschooled yet brilliant golfer. His story continues. I could talk about his artistic talent. But what I really want to say is: I admire Charlie most for his stunning ability to communicate with – to coin a phrase – 'all sorts and conditions of men' (well, persons). He is a quite remarkable person. He has had more life experience than we would have wished on anyone of his age, but he has consequently enormous resources and understanding which he has already used to good effect. I love to say that he drives me crazy from time to time but I guess that goes along with the privilege of being regarded as part of the family. And that is how much I love you Charlie. I want to toast to you on your twenty-first but I also want to say – go for it Charlie, because you have so much to offer.

Cleo also recently wrote a lovely piece for this book:

> Charlie – the 'golden boy'!
>
> Such glorious memories of Charlie, Layla, Matt and my girls in Wales – where they had the freedom to run, sing, 'dance' and laugh together – will always be with me.
>
> Charlie had a brilliant future ahead of him and we were aware of both his sporting and artistic talents.
>
> When he was diagnosed with MS we were profoundly shocked and then whilst coming to terms with no more football, we watched his artistic talent progress and flourish. Charlie amazed me then, and even more now, with his graceful acceptance of a more sedentary life. Of course, he can be annoying (aren't we all?) but *never* have I heard him complain. He has great strength and in many ways is a great example to us all.
>
> Charlie and I travelled the world together when he was in the rehab centre – obviously in our imagination – but we had fun and I am sure he does and will succeed in many ways, however different.
>
> Charlie, I love you.
>
> Cleo

Cleo's ex-husband Geoff decided to become my honorary godfather just because he loves me so much, and truly he has always been by my side. He is one of those who was convinced I would become a professional footballer. I really relate to his true Irish character and he always seems on fire. I am a younger version of him in many ways. We have in common a certain style with the ladies, going with the flow towards them with almost no restriction. However, he is still a father image, without the downsides. For instance, when he was man-sitting me, he would have let me smoke inside the house when it is frowned upon by my parents.

Their daughter is my age and has been a very close friend since primary school. As we lived on the same street, we used to catch the bus to school together. When we were both about 13, our families went on holiday to the south of France together at my godmother's chateau. One evening, she had an argument with her mum and ran away into the nearby woods. It caused havoc.... Since then, this dynamic and gorgeous girl has become highly successful, working for an investment bank. Through her, I keep in touch with a bunch of school friends. It is great to still have that social circle but I must admit that sometimes I get jealous of her professional and social successes. She was travelling on my birthday so couldn't celebrate with me. Here is the message she sent:

> Happy birthday my darling Charlie. I love you my brother. You are a light in my life and the best person I know. So sad not to be with you on your day – looking forward to celebrating middle age with you. All the love in the world – Lucy xxxx

Anna is one of our greatest friends, and also went to school with us. She was a wonderful actress and eventually became an amazing photographer. We have so much respect for each other. She is one of the very few who sticks with me as a friend, accepts me for who I am without judgement and does not get irritated as most people do. She makes me feel so comfortable when we are out together, giggling at my strange ways with people and making sure they feel comfortable as well. She holds a great power in being able to control me. For instance, she easily stops me when I am going over the top with ladies. It is probably because she doesn't mind if I go a bit wacky that she can handle my most bizarre ways. She is so cool; I love her and am proud to know her. Mum would not hesitate to ask her to look after me sometimes because she trusts her so much and knows how she can care for me. She started to help me on my art course and quickly revealed herself as the best art assistant I have ever had, because she knows me really well and respects my creativity, and also because she is so creative too. Her mere presence helps me to produce the best I can do. I feel so safe and free with her, it helps me draw good lines and choose good colours. Moreover, her natural beauty and joy are also a great inspiration. Therefore, I thought it would be a really good idea to ask her to help me write about art in this book, hoping I can inspire her as much as she inspires me.

Here are her words of wisdom and a poem she wrote for my fortieth birthday. My sister and my cousin Jay gathered my life into an amazing collage of pictures and words for that birthday; it is truly representative of my journey in life until this moment in time.

> Words of wisdom:
> Always know how much you make me smile.
>
> Poem:
> It's a certain person's birthday,
> A big one, yes, it's true,
> We want to celebrate him
> (and maybe get drunk too).
> With a beard to rival ZZ,
> And baby blues so bright,
> He's a special kind of character,
> Now ladies, please don't fight.
> The silver-tongued cavalier,
> Is how he's often known,
> Or maybe he's Charlie to you,
> When he calls you on the phone.
> He's an artist, first and foremost,
> And a writer with great gifts,
> He's a ninja on the chess board,
> Just don't offer him a spliff.
> He speaks to all and sundry,
> Much to his parents' disdain,
> He's the king of his community,
> And forever may he reign.
> So, yes, he drives some wheels now,
> But he's still the man to be,
> With his lust for life and warmest heart,
> It's the inimitable, CB.
> (So much love,
> From your pal, A)

Another crucial relation is my parents' very good friend Zoe, who became my very good friend too. She is a glorious lady with the beauty of a princess and she is very generous, in every way. I especially appreciate her listening skills. She would take me out, really caring for my struggles. She would give me loads of tips to help me deal with my parents and remind me how I could care for them better. She really knows how to stroke my heart. Because she understands me so well, I asked her to write a contribution to this book for me. Here is her letter, as a snapshot of my life:

> Dearest Charlie,
>
> You've asked me to write a short piece to go into your book. I'm honoured to do that, and I hope writing it as a letter will be alright.
>
> I haven't seen your book yet, but I know it's about your life so far and I think it is a marvellous achievement to have written it. I expect it will be full of all kinds of stories about how things have been for you – funny, touching, sad, happy, even lurid stories, just like the best books are! You've already had a life with so much packed into it – far more than most people who never have to deal with the sorts of things you've had to take on.
>
> I remember you as a clever little boy with such a lot of energy and charm. You were quite shy, but always friendly and with a wonderful gift at football, which you worked at really hard. When you first became ill it must have been very frightening for you, and deeply upsetting. I have never heard you complaining. You have never been self pitying. You have always maintained the most amazing zest for friendship and for every aspect of life. I expect the book will have a few stories about where this energy led you to in your twenties, when you were beginning to really feel the effects of the MS and its disturbance. You had as wild a time as anyone could, sometimes putting yourself in quite scary situations, always with an eye for the girls – who always had eyes for you too, you were/are so gorgeous to look at! It was as if you were defying the illness, and doing it with huge courage, even if often without enough care for yourself.
>
> You are also an artist. Your work has been interfered with by illness but you have a wonderful eye for line and colour and a freedom to experiment that has given your work a real presence. I know how glad my daughters are to have your portrait of their father on their walls. It's a lovely, warm image and it was a very kind idea of yours to make it.

> When I think of you, courage and generosity of spirit are what come most immediately to my mind. You've never given up on your interest in the world around you and your wish to contact other people. I have huge respect for this and for you. I just wish you'd never had to battle so hard. You have always been ambitious, with aspirations to make a real difference and win respect and attention. I hope you know how much you've succeeded already in doing this – and there's clearly even more to come, with this book!
>
> I know you only want a short piece from me. I hope this is about right. The main thing is how lovable you are. And this comes from me with great love.
>
> Zoe

My parents' friends, just like my parents themselves, are all soul-giving and soul-embracing. These are very rare qualities that can go deeper than the ocean. It is knowing when and how to be fully available and empathetic, while being true to oneself and explaining clearly and softly one's own limits. It is an ability to listen to others' feelings and expressing their own, while putting things into perspective, and bringing good humour to the bigger picture. Not only do they care for others, these people can also thrive in the party with bubbling energy, creativity and humour. Huberistically, I feel that I am part of that soul-giving group of people and that is giving me the confidence to deal with life's worries and hassles.

Chapter 3

Glories of mental and love ventures

Jesus Christ saga

Summer '96 – I was 19 and had spent 2 years struggling between school and hospitals with a new state of mind and life, under heavy medication and discovering other get-out clauses such as drugs, sex, art and music. I hadn't been diagnosed with bipolar yet but my mental state was getting out there. Coming back from art college, I was so high that I was showing off my pieces of art and portraits in many local cafés. Furthermore, I could not stand being closed in; I was desperate to escape my situation. I was behaving literally like a wild animal as soon as I felt trapped, with a super strength helping me fly away from any locked door or wall.

After a short life in football, where I was flying around the pitch, feeling trapped became an obsession. I was jumping over garden fences like a London fox. One morning I woke up, switched on the TV and saw a programme on Jesus Christ: that was me!!! Life had crucified me! But I was born again and felt exalted. I laid down on the grass in the garden in a JC crucifix position, my arms wide open and my legs crossed. I was empowered and saved. Diving into a Jesus Christ halo became the only way to feel calm. My mum called the GP and another miracle happened – the GP came! In this country you actually need to be Jesus Christ to have a GP visit you!

The GP felt I should be sectioned. My mum couldn't stand the idea. For readers who are not aware of these mental health administration delicacies, a person who is in danger to him or herself or to other people can be sectioned under the Mental Health Act, which means being put away in a psychiatric unit against their will and for an unknown amount of time. This would drive anyone crazy, would it not? Moreover, being sectioned gives an official status and puts a lunacy label upon people which they will never escape from even when they are back to 'normal'. My mum was – and still is – fighting for my rights like a tiger, otherwise I would probably today be behaving like a lobotomised tired man, trapped in that disabled and dangerous status until the end of my life, unable to feel responsible and just scaring everyone. Thank God for my mum! Therefore she hid me from the mental health sectioners and took me with her to a friend's house, spending a full day in a dark room to calm me down and explain that being sectioned by the mental health services would ultimately be the worst place for me.

Mum managed to convince me to go voluntarily to a mental health hospital, which is the only alternative to being sectioned. I was sent to a psychiatric unit, and that was my church. I was so glad to be able to bless everyone around and to save souls. I was over-elated, more than I'd ever felt before, clearly in the power of the universe and all its beings. Trying to control me, doctors gave me heavy drugs. I was so high already that it didn't have much effect. I was still the one and only Jesus Christ, happy to show everyone that I could walk on water when there was spillage of water on the bathroom floor. That was such blasphemy that they drugged me even more and I started to become a different man.

I was no longer dazzling, my self was leaving me, I felt dead to the world, and I was becoming vulnerable to my other very dysfunctional companions in the ward. A gay guy with AIDS was chatting me up. I got beaten up by three nurses who would not let me go for a piss. I never understood the full reason why it happened. My mum decided to take me away and we stayed at home until she managed to get an appointment at our local hospital – where my brother and I were born – where they decided to keep me. There I met the Lord and Warrior from South London. They told me I was the Officer of the area. It confused me at first but then I remembered that, when I was a kid with my father in the car, we stopped in a garage, and I told a rioting group to *hush* and they went away. So everything was making sense and being the Officer took me higher than ever. Or maybe they gave me that status because I was giving them cigarettes??? Or maybe not! However, I felt everyone was loving me so much, whether I was Jesus Christ, the Officer or Charlie Bacchus.

I was there for three weeks and had a good time. A lady in there thought she was a prostitute and wanted to have a shag in the toilets. I knew that Jesus Christ wouldn't have had any problem sleeping with her even though she was a prostitute, but clearly I was not attracted to her – I have my values and I know I can get much better. That was probably a sign that they had managed to bring me down a great deal and I was not that crazy any more. Or is it that this person saved me in bringing my consciousness back? After all, I know that after a period of time they found the right medication and managed to stabilise me on chemicals, which I have been on ever since. It does seem to work really well as I have never been threatened with being sectioned again (sure, I have been close to it though). Thank you, Professor Michael Kopelman, for finding the right drug.

But I also felt very very low. All my friends had gone on their year off. I was just moping around in bed, with no energy. For about two years I was taken by these regular low points called depression that could last for about three months. What would you expect from a young football champion having been struck down with illness when all he wanted to do was score goals upfront? Although my life force was leaving me, I never considered suicide and I was not angry. Actually, anger does not take hold of me at all, whatever happens. My existence was crucial because of all this love around and inside me, and also because of a top, structured education mixing creativity, freedom and order. I was aware and highly appreciative of my parents' hard work to give their kids a future. Even when I was deeply depressed, I could feel an inner strength nurtured by this family love and solid guidance and I could tell my future was a great one. For instance, I remember a letter from my sister who was in university, telling me she would always be there for me. That touched me beyond anything. My brother Matt's presence was also crucial to me feeling protected and full of beans. Moreover, a new confidence was arising with the explosion of my sex life.

I was labelled bipolar and had regular medication, counselling sessions, psychiatric check-ups and a worried family. Fortunately, the depression didn't last and mania came into force, with the conviction I could live my life to the fullest. This was not so easy for the family, but they managed to accept the man I was becoming.

Art, ladies and dope

End of summer '96 – all my friends were going back to normal life, football and work but I didn't have a job, just a daily dose of medicine to keep me sane. I went to an art course in Kentish Town where I felt like I was alive again. I made new friends and was able to be really creative again, especially as I also discovered the joys of drugs and sex. My mind found a new balance with this mix of legal and illegal drugs, plus art and sex – all a perfect fit for my manic personality. Within a year of a new-found creativity, I got the first and only diploma of my life. Fortunately, I soon became the silver-tongued cavalier. Don't need a diploma for that, just to be very good with the ladies....

The weed-smoking all started with my sister and her friends when I was about 13. It was her sixteenth birthday, early on an evening at home, with about ten boys and girls from school. The boys already knew about marijuana and passed some spliffs around. After a few puffs, I felt uplifted, extremely relaxed, happy and naughty, since my parents were downstairs. Then I knew what high meant and I loved both that intense inner feeling and being disobedient. I was not too attracted by the world of drugs then, just occasionally for fun like any other teenager. My favourite place was still the football pitch, playing for a little league, and my aspiration was to play in a big team like Tottenham Hotspur.

However, when I got MS I fell into the weed-world big time, also encouraged by the fact that it was supposed to be good for people with MS. But it wasn't – actually it's rather terrible for my condition where MS and mania are very closely linked. Weed just led me to mania straight away, where I felt really good, loving myself and the world even more, which was beneficial considering the dark cloudy place I was in. Smoking would lighten and brighten up those clouds. As I wasn't into sports any more, but rather with arty people, drugs were a normal way of life, opening up our brains and bodies, allowing us to relax completely and make utopia a reality. Sex was the obvious following activity, whether it was in the park, in the toilets or in my or their bedroom. We had loads of fun. That is how my gangster sex life started.

I started to hang on to the belief that everyone should live their life as if it's their last day on earth, every single day. To others this might be an incorrect way to live one's life, as we all have responsibilities. Except ME! Taken care of and labelled 'un-abled'. This developed a self-centred *carpe diem* attitude in me that transformed my life completely. It was the only way to cope, coming from a feeling of being lost with myself, not able to build a career nor to fit into any of this society's boxes. I was smoking an ounce of weed a week and I was a sexual bandit with no responsibilities. I wasn't even wearing condoms until my parents bought them for me; I don't know if any or many children were brought to life … Living with my lovely family in a Victorian house in a beautiful 'safe' area gave me enough security and safety to allow myself complete freedom. At the time, I still had good balance with my legs, so no one would have guessed that I was sick.

My girlfriends were happy to bring me some weed and other drugs such as cocaine. Mixing both would take us to the higher level.

I could have 7 ladies in one week and another 6 available as I counted having 13 affairs going on at once. The girls just wanted a very good shag and didn't mind being considered as a one-off or one of many. Because I know how to satisfy a woman.… As mentioned before, my erection could last for ever because I could not ejaculate. This would give me plenty of time to understand exactly what they desired. Like my football skills, this was like a God-given gift to me, along with my charisma and good looks. They all fitted together and added to my manic personality.

I was feeling like a demi-god, enjoying giving pleasure as much as receiving it. After a love session, they would fall asleep and often miss the next day at work. I enjoyed looking at them asleep after a long session of passion, feeling fully content for both of us and proudly knowing they would always be back for more. It was not just physical; giving a lady a huge orgasm is crucial and very emotional for me. I was feeling so close and linked to them, on an intimate and creative journey to the best state of mutual gratitude, and gratitude towards the whole universe. It was definitely a pure spiritual venture that would bring deep thoughts and chats.

Learning about the female species' specifications was a real joy. I was in love with them all but I would make sure they would not fall for me, even though they did. At times, keeping several relationships going would make me feel guilt-ridden and drive me crazy, so I much preferred to keep my freedom and pride by flagging up my single status. I would never give out my phone number; they knew where I lived anyway. Of course, I would never ever be disrespectful to them, rude or violent. After the action and a bit of rest, I would always ensure that they understood I was not available for a romantic relationship, just sex and friendship; being a polygamist would not be respectful to them nor to my own values. They would try to get through to me by getting even more sexual, even ready for anal sex, which I appreciated of course. But I always kept a respectful attitude, enjoying their company, listening to them and always remembering their qualities. Having so many sexual partners definitely made me feel like a real man. MS was not that scary any more.

My mother understood that, even though she didn't know about the majority of my ladies. She was polite to the few girls that I brought home and kind enough to serve them a nice cup of tea in the morning. However, she asked me to stop treating the house like a brothel. 'I am not your Madam', she said, as I was bringing ladies home without building any relationships. Fortunately for her, I wasn't also bringing into my 'boudoir' all the dodgy people I was dealing with.

To please my mum, I had to live my sexual gangster's and druggy life outside the family home. I would go to the ladies' homes, which was much better, as it often turned into orgies. There are also loads of various secret places where you can make love. When there is an urge, one can always find a location to release it. I wouldn't even mind the girls' weird mental states, being mental myself. I would let it slide, just like my penis in the punani. All pussies would give me joy. A crazy one could be great fun and bring even greater sex. Actually, we were all nymphomaniacs. When the reputation got out there, ladies came to me ten a penny. I was using them like Kurt Cobain did cocaine. Fortunately, I didn't die of it.

I got mature enough to become a bit more responsible and not forget the condoms. I had so many of them I could sell one for a pint. I would also trust my internal feelings when a girl wasn't sexually healthy. I can usually feel when a woman is carrying an STD; I get a cold warning sensation from her aura and her eyes. A few sad anecdotes confirmed this instinct that avoided me getting AIDS. I wish I could develop that clarity on other human mishaps.

I met quite a few unclean girls too but didn't always have time to find out, lost in the sexual parade and then lost inside their cunts. The scent of their huge orgasms would hide the dirty other ones. My long-lasting erection would avoid me going down there and dealing directly with the bad smell.

Luckily, my pattern for the ladies was good looks, good eyes and good eyebrows, good education, character and charm (I admit I'm a bit posh even though I'm a rebel). These qualities would open the door for a real good shag and eventually, later, to a proper relationship. However, at that time I was too busy tasting the fruits of the world to be able to build relationships.

My parents would not allow me to smoke weed at home and got fed up with the heavy habit of weed-smoking, especially as it proved to accelerate my symptoms of mania. Truly, it pushed me to discover the female form without any boundaries. For most men, ejaculation calms them down to the point that they feel sleepy, but in my case the finale would never come. Therefore, sex pushed me on and on to a higher plane and I could shag for ever.

Hoping to get me more focussed and take me away from the druggy people in the art world, my parents made sure I was in a good college and signed me up to do design studies. I had a beautiful teacher there who fortunately knew about my condition (I have never been shy about it). Her beautiful derrière was such a visual delight! And she had a great personality as well. I knew it was improper to touch her but it was so appealing I could not help myself slapping that sexy lady on her derrière. SILLY ME! She could tell I was on a strange high and she was kind enough not to make a big fuss about it. She also knew I was not very happy doing design studies and encouraged me to go to another college to learn typography. It was also probably a way for her to get rid of me from the course.

I would have much preferred to go back to a proper art college and I still feel resentful for that. My college was an incredible place, as all the ladies were absolutely stunning, ticking all the right boxes. I felt that studying typographic design was quite boring, but I enjoyed life-drawing so much; I love seeing the gloriousness of women's bodies and they obviously enjoyed my attention. It regularly drove us insane and into beautiful lovemaking.

Making love is like producing the most beautiful piece of art. Inspiration can come from anywhere – images, feelings, fantasies. Just like the form of women's beautiful bodies, auras, scents, or any kind of look they give, especially when they're happy and excited. Creation has no boundaries, just like my sexual nature. It starts small with an idea or an image that arouses the freedom of self and grows with each gesture in a self-nurturing way. Each new piece of art or new girlfriend is a mark in one's life history.

Of course, I have always been a lover not a hater; however, making love glorified my existence and increased my sense of being high on life. That was a gangster's paradise. I kept this radiant attitude that transformed my life from a sportsman to a lover, and also broke the boundaries of my illness in many different ways. Satisfying the ladies became a way to challenge the curtailment of the disease, feeling virile, strong and powerful. It was the key to the vitality of my existence. I was lucky that my MS was a hidden illness. My impossibility to ejaculate was keeping me at it for hours. My hard-on couldn't die and I quickly became the Orgasmic Master.

The only problem was that I could not cum inside the ladies and would often finish it myself with a good wank, but believe it or not, ejaculation would not even bring me any orgasm. The girls usually loved to swallow my cum and many told me it had a really good taste, which made me happy again. I never felt sleepy after such long lovemaking; the Taoists say it is because I kept my sperm inside my body. Strangely, the first obvious symptom of my MS has quickly become my greatest strength and happiness. Giving a lady an orgasm is my own orgasm. It is the best way to feel completely alive. Strangely, being fully there for the other makes oneself feel one's own existence is complete. I had never imagined that I would become a sex addict or a sex god but that is how I was, softly killing my illness' sadness.

It should have been enough to make me feel whole but it rarely solidified into a proper relationship and I still needed to escape my condition, as I was looking for drugs all the time. I can see now that I didn't want to feel real. The number of girls and drugs were never enough; the more I had the more I wanted. My life was definitely out of the fire into the frying-pan. I had lost direction and control and I didn't care about my health nor my dignity – that disappeared with the number of ladies I was bedding.

Even though I was a sex god, I could feel inside that my life was not going anywhere and I needed the drugs to flee from that pathetic feeling. Heavy sex was not enough to hide my condition from myself. I thought that drugs would hide my own despair. Weed and coke took me to crack and heroin. Fortunately, even with my addictive personality, I never got into those so-called heavy drugs because I didn't feel their effect much. Crack is only one quick rush and I was more attracted to the dodgy people around it than to the poison itself. Their crazy sad lives made me feel a bit better about myself. I knew that my family would stop me from falling into the bad trap they were in. I was definitely attracted by their wild ways with no boundaries and they gave me the impression that they would still find balance in their strange lives. Oddly, I never felt the effects of heroin, probably because of my basic happy mood. It seems that heroin is only for very depressed people. I still don't understand why people would spend so much money on that stuff. I just smoked it once and never took the risk of shooting it in my veins as I was aware of all the dangers, AIDS and addiction.

I clearly knew that I was living an insane life but I didn't care, even though my entourage was telling me that my way of life was particularly dangerous for my condition. Hearing that, it would just push me into the deeper trap of getting higher and just forgetting about it, thinking I had nothing to lose. The worst things I could lose would be my close family's love, which would never happen anyway, and life. I don't think I have ever been scared of dying. For me death is just one part of this journey we are all living. I have also never wished to die. I don't really care about all this, just need to enjoy what is left here for me, and keep on sharing and giving.

Only 15 minutes' walk away from home was a drug pick-up zone. I was enjoying pulling my head off and mingling with all kinds of people, until I couldn't move. The only thing I could remember was my parents' phone number and I was not ashamed to call them and ask them to come and pick me up. When my desperate mum arrived, I would feel both relieved and guilty, like a little boy. I was hanging on to the idea that Mum loved me and my art, and things would get better because I have a magic family.

Mum's poem written during that heavy period of time:

I am who I am because I am
This powerful talented beautiful young man
Struggling for identity
The soul within crying out loud
I am who I am because I am invincible I can cure my pain

Let me in to say how beautiful you are
The wolves see it too
Come they say be free with us
Because we are vulnerable too
And we want to collect you into our tribe
Not because we believe in you
But because we need you to survive
We need your money to get the stuff
To hide our pain
And who is to blame for our shame
The underworld is beckoning us
To share a brief moment
Of elation and fame
I'm Jesus Christ I say
As they laugh and collude
With the demon's standing by
Ready to blow the mind
I am who I am I say
I do not care who you are
Because I am free and need not care
Millionaire for the day
The people I love will take the pace
And pay
Pay for the debt
Of aggression and challenge
The elation and the drive
The tramp-like apparition
The beggar the drunk
The desperation to belong
The rejection the frustration
Of friends who once stood by
Long time gone
Six months down the line
The depth of despair
The controlling drugs
The sadness and the blame
For shattered lives
I love him but the
Exhaustion and the pain
I am who I am because I am I say
But where have you gone

Within this frame
Of isolation and loss
Mobility gone
Crawling up from the abyss
A repeated pattern
Year after year
You remain beautiful still
I am who I am I say
But to whom
They have all gone
By my motherhood

Seduction course

Looking girls in the eye, engaging them in conversation and, moreover, listening to what they have to say – that is crucial to attract and entice a lady. Engaging in a listening manner is the first trick, just asking them about themselves, showing interest in their identity and their activities. You cannot just rush in and express your physical feelings for them immediately, of course. My second trick is complimenting them about their eyebrows, which is becoming a bit more personal and more original. Eyebrows above beautiful eyes are among some of my favourite interests in women. Everyone looks into the eyes without noticing that the shape of eyebrows is a very important piece of art/part of the face. Furthermore, they show how much a woman is taking care of herself. And that really gets me going, in a huge manner!

Then you can compliment their lips and how each feature of their face sits together as one.

At this point, they are usually getting a lot more sexified and you can find out if they are married. It is crucial information before moving to the next level. Their honesty usually breaks the final barriers, as they have made a promise in front of God. In my case, it is rather good news to have a husband in the loop as they won't be looking for commitment. Or, if they have a partner or are too up tight to deepen the relationship, I don't waste any more time chatting them up. I wouldn't show any frustration, hurt or resentment; I'd be charming about it and I'd go around the corner and get another girl.

Their reaction to the husband question shows me how to express the love I am going to give them. When I feel the husband subject is a delicate issue to bring up and makes them frown, I know that they just need some of my demi-godly touch and never-ending erection. If they don't want to mention the husband at all, it means the gates are wide open with no barriers. Those ladies with a frustrating husband usually want rough sex, i.e. going anal. They want to feel the pain because they have a painful relationship. I am aware I can hurt so I would always be careful and encouraging, as delicate as possible. I would ask them if they want to use gel; some would refuse just to feel it even harder. They like my style, which is a fun pain that they can control and will usually bring lots of pleasure.

Even though I am aware that I am a bit cunning, bringing a red rose to a date shows purity, romance and kind intentions. Even if I am not looking for a relationship, the red rose puts me in a different light. The girl may not know what she desires, therefore the rose dramatises the moment and adds that 'je ne sais quoi' that will entice her in. And she will keep it as a souvenir of the beautiful love-making, knowing that its thorns may hurt. That is the story of love.

Another way to get girls into my house is to offer to show them my artwork, but we manage to have sex even before I have a chance to present anything to them. I always give them a piece of my art, rather than my phone number. They leave satisfied with the memory of this creative and passionate evening. Knowing where I live, they would sometimes come around to catch me. Or, as mentioned before, in my early twenties, I would enjoy going around with my artwork in a portfolio to show my art off all over. That would definitely attract ladies' attention and get me into many debaucheries. I was at the top level of my tantric sex period, as my erection would last for hours.

Tantric sex

It can take a lifetime for very open-minded men to learn about tantric sex. Tantric sex is the art of everlasting bodily love, by knowing to postpone the ejaculation and keeping an erection for hours. I am grateful my illnesses gave me this natural ability. How many people know that love is most enjoyable, fulfilling and healthy without an orgasm?

Actually, generating and keeping the semen inside strengthens the man's energy. Ask old Far Eastern gentlemen how they are taught not to ejaculate for nine times in a row. Keeping their sperm inside is not only a technique to make the lady happy and allow her to come in her own time, or to show her own sexual prowess; it is a physiological way to build up male inner vigour and consequently keep really healthy. It is such a tool for longevity that in ancient China sex and love was an important branch of medicine. Besides regulation of ejaculation, *The Tao of Love* also explains the importance of female satisfaction and that 'orgasm and ejaculation are not necessarily one and the same thing' (Jolan Chang, *The Tao of Love and Sex: The Ancient Chinese Way to Ecstasy*).

For me, all this felt just so natural, not only using my penis, also my hands, my tongue and my whole body. It is so beautiful and easy to let instinct lead the way and discover the new erogenous regions of her body. It is an exciting game to find out which are the woman's favourites and even to discover together new orgasmic zones. Therefore, I realised that giving pleasure without using my dick was often much more dazzling for both me and the lady than just rubbing and pumping into her hole. This is why 'you've got to go for the clit, not just the slit!' (that's what my last girlfriend said – she's got such a large clit …). Giving the lady a huge orgasm makes you feel the proudest man on earth! Moreover, bringing the lady to such a cosmic feeling can lead to further places or dimensions, such as anal or spiritual.

Ladies tell me that most men don't actually know where the clitoris is or how to handle it. If you're very insightful, careful and engaging with the lady, you can tell when you are hitting the spot, as you delicately rub her, with the change of her face and her moans. The nipples also become more erect. The clit is first hidden under a lot of skin on top of the woman's peachy pussy, waiting to be softly awoken, so it can grow with excitement and further arouse the whole zone, including the vagina of course. This is one of the reasons why it is quite improper to go directly into the vagina when it is not awoken. Bringing in a little bit of laughter also helps the arousing.

The key is to make the lady feel completely relaxed. The funny thing is that a lady's clitoris is a male's penis, just as erectile but much smaller and fragile. You must be very gentle with the lady's most sensitive spot. It is such a delicate tiny flower concealed to protect itself from nasty rushing impatient visitors, so much so that some girls don't even know where it is, or worse, some have never got off to it. It is such an exciting and empowering feeling to show a lady her most intimate point and teach her how to explore the joy she can get from it.

You can start by licking or tickling her thigh or nipples or *nombril* (belly button in French) to smooth her into a relaxed and abandoned motion. Then you can move in to gently lick the area and allow the clit to become active. In following the girl's moans and your own instinct, you will finally get there, feel it becoming bigger and bigger and get the whole zone aroused. If for some reason you cannot find it, just ask the girl to show you where it is. Most women would be too shy about their private garden to be able to ask directly where to go. You should make a gentle motion around it and above it, but again never be too rough on it as it can get easily hurt. For some women the clit orgasm can take a long time. Never give up on it because your persistency and consistency will make her feel so wanted and cherished that she will eventually let go of her intellectual protection and defences to finally free herself and come heavily and joyfully.

You will feel if the girl prefers a quick clit orgasm or if your intimacy, the clit's excitement and the whole moisterisation are encouraging you to go down to the vagina. There is an even bigger deeper stronger orgasm waiting there. Basically, it is waiting for the ultimate and glorious unification of two people coming together and exploding with love. However, as we said, starting with the clit is electrolysing the glorious delicacies of the vulva. It also encourages the woman to tighten her inner muscles, which is going to get the deeper orgasm to come. Again, if she does not know that herself, you can suggest it to her. She is often so taken away by the whole thing that she sometimes hardly concentrates on what is happening down there.

Women, listen up now: you have so many muscles inside your secret garden. You should exercise them as a daily gardening routine to prepare them for lovemaking. Getting the woman to tighten and contract her muscles also keeps your erection on. It is definitely worth being patient and waiting for the woman's hidden paradise to be ready for exploration. So, all men reading this, please learn! Getting a woman off with your tongue rather than your dick is really empowering and brings new sexual realms.

Moreover, it is also extremely good for your health, as the oestrogens liberated by the female orgasm boost immunity, repair tissues and protect against heart disease. These are scientific facts published by the New England Research Institute in 2010. Experts are recommending men go down there twice a week to keep healthy.

Now, when you have a very powerful erection which can last for hours, it opens the door for many many things; for example, it allows you to satisfy several women together. I could use my hand, my tongue and my dick with two or three different women at once. It is even more exciting! Usually I would have had glorious sex with them individually beforehand, and, as they would always want more, I would try to make a threesome happen. It wasn't hard at all to convince them, as I realised a threesome was quite a common fantasy for women. They enjoy discovering their own female organs and sexuality in one another. It is so beautiful to have these stunning beautiful naked women wrapped around me, swelling, moaning and screaming. Sometimes they would enjoy it so much that they may have even thought they were becoming lesbians.

These Tantric sex times were probably the most glorious. It is such an empowering joy to get a woman to find out about her own femininity and her own self.

Dirty sex

Of course, the art of silver-tongue cavaliering is only possible when the secret garden's scents are attractive to the man. I would never allow a smelly stinky and sticky cunt to come my way. Nature is so good to give us this efficient warning about a woman's health and salubriousness. Unfortunately, too many girls don't take care of themselves.

Another good spot is the zone between the anus and the vagina. It is scientifically called the perineum. It can get the lady off big-time and helps relax the anal area in case you want to try to get there.

I have never ever been disappointed with a girl, first because I instinctively pick up the good vibes, second because I always satisfy them. Third, I consider myself a gentleman and therefore would never ever dis or harm a woman; I respect them all and appreciate their qualities. It would be useless and sad if I were to dig at them; I would never do or say anything that may be negative for myself or anyone else. I am one of the good guys.

My reputation spread among the elite community, starting with a classy local male hood who was asking me to chat women up for him. It was easy for me to convince any lady and her friend to come out up to the city with my rich mates and I. Money and alcohol would do the job, as I would seduce her girlfriend and she would end the evening with the rich stockbroker. This became a juicy business for a little while, as these guys would show their gratitude with a nice lump of cash.

During those sexual champion/obsession days, many elite women also led me into some kind of prostitution. My reputation had got out in the world of posh ladies desperate for a good shag, as they knew they would never get disappointed with me. I would get a call from an unknown woman paying a cab to drive me to a beautiful hotel, sometimes to a beautiful countryside mansion, where she would be waiting for me, half naked, sexy and desperate for my killer erection. They were mostly rich married women in their forties, whose wealthy husbands were not able to satisfy them. Those banker guys are probably too obsessed with money-making or power-growing to be able to fuck. But part of their power would be to marry sexy princesses. They would always be beautiful, with a nice ass and a delectable scent to them.

The upper-crust females always know how to take care of themselves: shaved pussy and ass, most beautiful perfume all over their body, softest skin in the whole world. They would also take care of me with a beautiful meal and good wine. Some were idiotic enough to say they wanted to divorce their millionaire husbands and marry me just because of a good night's shag. I felt complimented but would never ever go that way. Getting involved in a divorce is not my style. I just offered to shag them again but, as I had so many ladies at the same time, I was not that available, which raised the auction. Sometimes they would go up to £10,000 for a month-long shagging. I would usually take £1,000 for an hour and could get up to £3,000 to go anal and get really dirty, or to invite other women around. The suitcase of money would be waiting for me on my arrival, managed by my accountant who would put it in a private account and make sure it was well spent. *Really*!!! My Mum thinks this is absolute bollocks and doesn't believe it, but I know it's true.

I would sometimes ask the princesses to put the money into charities. I felt like I had a fantastic job, as I had to be very well organised to please everyone and keep it very private, especially for my parents. I didn't even think of paying myself to get independence from them; I wanted to stick by my family that I love so much. My dirty secrets would help me take poorer ladies out and pay for hotels to avoid bringing them home. It would also pay for coke and weed of course, sometimes Es (Ecstasy), not only for me and my girls but also for the extra-cool addicts' community of the area. I was doing it for the fun, to blow the cash away and especially to be part of this superfly underground world of dope fiends. I knew it was wrong but I really needed to escape my own ill body and brain, my own bourgeois world and these over-rich princesses' fake existences.

I liked to think about myself as Robin Hood, taking from the rich to be able to give back to the poor. We were all hanging out in the peace garden next to the church where I got involved in various misdemeanours that could have cost me my life. For instance, I told a big black guy that his Rolex was fake, and he just wanted to kill me. Strangely, I never got addicted myself, especially as I never got high on my own supply and I was more interested in the people than in the coke's effect. To me it is not more effective than a strong coffee. The princesses loved it though, as they were not used to it and just wanted to get crazy. I much prefer weed, which is, unfortunately, so bad for me. However, I feel very fortunate that I never got addicted to any drug, even though I always tried to escape but never could. I still have an addictive personality because of my smoking and sexual habits.

Porn for Africa

In 1995 I met this South African guy who was accompanying Nelson Mandela in South London. We became mates, as we were both looking for ladies and I could advise him on the quality and the availability. We hit a fuse within each other and I got really interested in his work in Africa, where my parents were born. He talked about his mother's big charity, I told him about my mum's own charity and about the money I was making with the ladies. That is how the idea of a good partnership came up. I asked for paperwork to prove that my sexually funded money would be used properly. Now I know that it may have paid for some ANC arms and I do care about that. But at the time I was too young to bother. I was really happy to have found a positive use for my dirty activities.

From then on, it was even more exciting to raise my prices and the number of people involved. The price would start to go up for four-five-sevensomes and we raised the orgies up to 30 ladies!!! Sometimes the husbands would be invited to come, watch and wank but were not allowed to participate. People watching would make me feel very proud of my erection that would then grow in stature. When I realised how rich these people were, I decided to get the men to pay to be allowed to wank, up to £15,000.

These guys were mostly finance or business people, working every hour God had sent them and needing at least as much excitement as the huge power they had. Some came from upper upper-class families, very traditional English, very well-polished behaviour, from finishing schools. Some others were just very successful. It was easy to tell which ladies were very traditionally upper-class or just upper-class through the cash and power. They were all very beautiful outside and smelled really good, even inside their pussies. Their dress sense was amazing, their knickers were especially mind-blowing.

Some couples would also pay me to come with them to swinger clubs. It was incredible to be having so much sex with the richests. I got praised for having the best-tasting cum. I had to wank for that though, as I still never came once naturally during any of those orgies.

I also offered to do their portraits for £3,000, and £12,000 for a life drawing.

One guy offered a fortune to be allowed to participate in the orgy, but I turned him down. It felt so easy to dictate my own rules! I was treated as the Master of Ceremony, as a Roman prince organising his own bacchanals, as a sex dominator. Even though I enjoyed these powerful and rich people becoming my slaves, I never went into the dominatrix games. My fun was just to satisfy women and be the silver-tongued cavalier who would give money back to the poor.

It was like being the porn king some of my clients offered me to play in porn movies, but I never felt attracted to being a porn star. My inner pride told me not to go that way; I felt really good enough as a king in a private kingdom but didn't want to give it away to the public domain. I'd watched a lot of pornos as instruction manuals. My mum kept on throwing them away after they had given me some juicy ideas.

I was so proud of giving much pleasure, being worth so much money and giving food and water to so many poor people.

Maybe this whole Porn for Africa chapter of my life is a fantasy in my funny mind. I do feel it did happen though, and I definitely want to be very honest in this book – it needs to be.

During those years, I kept on with my usual girlfriends and family life. My family was a securing gate against the madness of wild sex. I was very good at hiding my crazy life from my loved ones. After 3 years and about 40 of those massive orgies, I met the woman of my dreams, fell in love and just wanted a steady relationship. Before I share with you this enrapturing true-love experience, I need to finish this dirty sex chapter with another mad episode. I am aware that these sexual stories can be very shocking, especially to my family. I am sorry if it hurts them but I really need to tell my own truth, even if some people may not believe it. It is such an exciting part of the life I have led!

Another side of sex

A few years after this chain-sex period, when I was about 28, I became fully aware of my growing MS symptoms, as I was now fully dependent upon my WS (walking stick). It was hurting so bad … I was still going to college, learning printmaking and photoetching. No love was floating around like it normally did. Doing a lot of drugs was keeping me away from depression, as well as keeping me away from too much sex. I became good friends with a black guy who played guitar on my high street for a living. He had understood my need for freedom and let me stay at his place for one night without expecting anything from me. We were doing crack together. I just needed another kind of escape but never really liked the flavour nor the effect, and it was affecting my erection a lot. I knew this guy was gay and couldn't come, just like me. He was very respectful to me and we just enjoyed each other's presence.

As he often went naked around his place, I had noticed his thick cock. One day we were so high, I don't really know how this happened, maybe I was just curious, I also wanted to please him – whatever, I just grabbed his cock and sucked it hard. I felt somehow alienated by this and didn't enjoy it much, but he was my mate and I was happy to please him. It was a new toy for my oral fixation but nothing as exciting and powerful as a lady's pussy. We tried further but my butt didn't like it at all. Our friendship grew with this little BJ favour I regularly gave him in exchange for a swift high that would allow me to forget my state of affairs for a little while. It was fine to know that I had this last port of call for a little crack fix and some kind of friendship, but I am definitely not gay and didn't feel attracted to that kind of existence.

However, later I deepened the homosexual experience with an English gay friend from college. He was more interested in me than me in him and had just a few drinks to offer. As usual I was quite open about my own sex life and had told him I could not come easily. He was quite proud to say it was easy for him to get people off. It was worth a try. Strikingly, his tongue had an amazing ability to work very quickly in a perfect coordination with his lips all over my cock to bring up all my cum. It was not only a question of motion, tightness and rhythm. What a muscled mouth he had! He made me come so much and so fast, more than I ever had: seven times in a row. It was even too much for him but he liked my crème caramel taste. I know from all the other girls that the taste of my cum is delectable. Probably its's because he's an actor and has a huge experience in the gay world. It was a great relief for me, more mental than physical, as I realised that my problem ejaculating was mainly a technical issue. However, these repetitive ejaculations didn't bring any kind of climax, not the slightest feeling of satisfaction … I did give him back the favour but I didn't like his flavour. So, this stayed a one-off experience. I much prefer my silver-tongue adventures with ladies to provide, enjoy and share their orgasms.

These smutty and dirty sex adventures versus true-love adventures clarified what I really wanted in love and sex: my favourite profile was and still is an older beautiful blonde with lovely legs, ass and breasts. A sharp brain and above all a deep giving soul is the key spiritual feeling that I want to get at first sight; this warm feeling from the heart and the mind goes beyond all. Sometimes it goes beyond reality as well and it is the expression of a kind of troubled spirit, just like mine.

Falling in love

The chain sex had stopped when I met my first proper girlfriend at a cricket match. Our eyes met and we felt a huge attraction to one another. She had a very powerful aura of success, maturity (she was definitely older than me) and fun. I gave her my number and was just hoping she would call me, but she didn't. I was daydreaming so much about her that I decided to go with another girl with the same first name, from a rich Ascot family, with a very strong education that didn't allow full sex. Plus, like most young girls, she didn't really know what she wanted with me.

When I got her text inviting me for supper at Café Rouge, I was expecting another complicated conversation. When I entered the café, I was very surprised to see the first girl with the same name who I had been fantasising about for a month. My dream was coming true: she was drinking champagne in a beautiful dress, all bubbly, obviously ready for anything. After three bottles of champagne, steak au poivre and my favourite desert, we decided to leave, and I then met her colourful sports car – *wow*, that fancy car was the cherry on the cake of this beautiful evening. It suited her so very well! We drove right into the next estate where she quickly gave me a BJ. She was an expert. Then we went to a late-night bar for cocktails and finished in my own boudoir at my parents'.

It was a crazy night of passion. The whole family was not surprised to meet her at the breakfast table. My dad recognised her from the cricket match. And here she was at once in my soul and part of the family. We went out for over a year, truly in love, learning to adapt to each other's needs. I was in my early twenties at the time and didn't really care about the age difference or any other limitations. But now I would know that such an incredible woman wants more than just fun. She realised she wanted to build a secure family and fell for a man who was supposed to give her all of that. I didn't mind her having an affair at first until I realised it was a very serious one. Our beautiful relationship broke up during a Christmas party. I was pissed and pissed off by this rival; I quickly started an argument with her that finished us off, pushing one another into the bushes.

Over ten years later she sometimes visits with a bottle of champagne and beautiful flowers for my mum. We are so happy to feel the same connection we had before, minus the passion and the sex. But I am definitely missing the passion and the sex very much, and her visits remind me of an old self that is not kicking anymore. I was feeling so sad after her first visit that I became really upset and disturbed a few days before her second visit. I behaved like a child, rebelling for nothing, whining, even taking money out of my father's wallet. My goal was just to escape with alcohol and dope. I managed to drink quite a lot of tequila before my mother found out. My dad was not only really upset at me, he was shocked and horrified. Luckily, he doesn't express it in a rough way. It seems that I act that way to provoke them and feel 'the rough' so I can feel alive and flee reality as well. Being cared for all the time is like being in a little bubble and it isn't real life. Anyway, after her visit, I was a lot calmer, as I felt understood and loved. She even offered for me to come and stay in her country house with her kids. We need to work that out.

Usually, every time there is a break-up, I keep on missing the woman a lot, forever, but I also recover very quickly because I don't want to be controlled by my feelings. I cannot stand the idea of a heartbreak and just look out for a new lady. The same night I break up can bring me another love!!! It could also push me back into chain sex. However, discovering real love for the first time had been so crucial to my soul that I didn't feel like going back to sex gangsterism. As a matter of fact, losing that first big love affected me a lot more than I first thought. Keeping that pain inside, unwilling to be aware of it certainly accelerated the development of MS, upsetting my affected neurones. Unfortunately, this neurological MS process was now 100 per cent confirmed by the docs.

More loves

Love in its glory brings feelings of pure contentment that are different from feeling high or the relief of an orgasm or an ejaculation (as I don't have orgasms). It is like reaching the pinnacle of my full identity which is just about love. I cannot resist telling you about some of these beautiful ladies. Most of those relationships would end up in a mutual fantasy-time in my boudoir. However, I did not have sex with all of them, even though various fantasies have always been very much alive within my mind! At the end of the day, I am not just sexually obsessed; I am more of a lover man and a dreamer, hoping to find *the* one, to build a relationship. Sometimes, I even dream of being polygamous: one woman for each day....

My ultimate love for a performer was probably the strongest love I have ever had in my existence so far. I would call her BIB (for Best in Bed), although my love for her still reaches far beyond the boudoir. I met her at the college where I was studying printmaking and she was teaching kids. Even though she was 20 years my senior, when our eyes met for the first time, we knew! A true love at first sight. Our souls connected first and then our bodies, in such a big way that we got engaged after two weeks. These connections are indescribable with words. I can just say it was turquoise, purple and yellow, my favourite colours that express for me all the powers from within. I felt happier with her than I ever felt with any other woman. I was already at the stage where I needed Viagra to keep my erection going and I would take four pills at once so she would make love to me all night, even when I was asleep and then again in the morning. I know the Viagra thing does not seem very healthy, but it helps with the MS symptoms (remember my nerves are deeply affected) and with the passion too! But I realise now that it must have damaged my neurologic system as well. Because we had such a good sex life and she had such a fantastic body – especially her 'derrière' – I couldn't see anything wrong with her. Her soul was staring at me in the third eye, right into my heart, watching and understanding my feelings and thoughts. I felt she completely got me: things were looking so perfect. Sadly, we couldn't live together because of the cash-flow situation and her kids, who didn't like me at all. I know now that we were both dreamers but that love was real.

My parents of course were not too happy with our engagement after two weeks. We were quite hurt when they took away the champagne that I had taken from them to celebrate our engagement. They thought the age gap was far too big but I was so happy with her that they did welcome her into the home and didn't put pressure on me. At first BIB didn't understand how much I needed to be taken care of and she started to dislike my mother who was still controlling my life, not in a malicious way but in a loving way. BIB didn't realise she also started to control me, as she was getting worried about me. She wanted me out of my parents' house but couldn't figure it out. Now I can see that she couldn't understand nor respect my parents' responsibilities towards me, but at the time I would rather have followed her everywhere and followed any mood she was in.

This triggered quite a lot of misunderstandings between me and my parents, as I thought they were doing it on purpose to break our relationship. Things got worse with a misadventure when I promised to give her something belonging to our family for her son's birthday party. But my mum disagreed and it became a big argument between the three of us. This was the beginning of the end of our love story. Moreover, we had an agreement that we would never cheat on each other and, with regret, I did.

I had been to a family party and one of my sister's girlfriends kissed me, out of nowhere, and everyone saw how much I enjoyed it and how we disappeared together for a while. Even my mum tried to stop me reminding myself that I was engaged. BIB had an intuition that something had happened there and managed to get it confirmed, so we had to split up. Interestingly, our relationship lasted a year and a day. I was very upset for quite a while, until now, years later. My heart still pines for her. I still refer to her as my ex-fiancée and I miss her very much. My soul tells me she is doing very well and we will meet sometimes in any of those worlds. I still miss the child I wanted to have with her.

I met my Norwegian princess at an adult college when I was still in love and involved with BIB. She was doing an acting course and I was doing printmaking. We met just outside the college, as we were both smokers. We got on straight away. She had just arrived from Norway, with her very blonde locks. I first fell for her blue eyes and then her delicious lips, and her incredible and dynamic character. As you know, my godfather is Norwegian and I had an opportunity to enjoy that culture with his son Frank. I like the way they are devoted to family and their character expresses this strong, healthy and charismatic Viking vibe. She was only 16, but we could talk as if we had known each other for centuries. She had a relationship going on so we didn't even have a snog. It was new to me to enjoy a woman's company knowing sex would not happen even though it was always on the cards. It was quite exciting but safe at the same time. I was feeling so free. My brain was even more activated because my phallus was not. She is a very intelligent lady and we have been able to keep that friendship up until now. Who knows its future? *I love her with all my heart*!

I met another beautiful lady on holiday; she was a single parent. Back in London, we hooked up on the Common close to where she was living, and love struck. She invited me to her friends' gatherings while her parents – who didn't like me – were looking after her child. I loved and respected her very much. She completed me in many ways. She knew how to have fun and made me so happy. However, as usual, the relationship could not go on. She knew I had other affairs and even if she accepted them, she didn't fancy a long-term relationship – neither did I. She officially left me because another of my girlfriends was making better money and she thought she would better suit me. I was quite shocked with that. Money should never play a part in love, but it always does. In this specific case, I believe she gave that reason because she could not find a better one. Maybe she had a new lover. However, she was quite right, as I stayed with that new woman for over two years and her cash was part of the joy.

I would like to introduce you to this amazing lady, Joy, who I met in a late-night bar. She was a blazing, dynamic lady with a top job, eight years older than me. She was amazed by the fitness of my cock because she'd never had that before. Our beautiful sex life looked like love, probably because she was not carrying any luggage into the relationship – no mental illness, no children, no husband, and she had some cash. It is the first and only time I had a kind of honeymoon, as she organised our trip to a Caribbean island. We spent nine days in a four-star hotel facing the sea. It reminded me of the Asian archipelago. It was raining to begin with, which encouraged our bed activities, and then we had fun in heaven on earth.

The people were quite different from the people in Asia though, less shy, and very friendly, sweet and polite. Really good people. They just made everyone feel at home. Actually, the beauty of this island is the people rather than the island itself, which is a bit dry and really poor. The divide between the tourists' and residents' lifestyle is massive. The money that comes in goes back to those big international corporations with nothing much left for the local people. Worse still, young local people prefer to sell drugs and sex to tourists than work; it's more fun and pays much better. It is sad to note that British TV has largely encouraged this kind of tourist culture.

Anyway, for somebody who loves to talk to everyone, this island was my paradise. I was chatting up the beautiful tourist ladies and that became a problem for my girlfriend who started controlling me. We had a few arguments and were finally both happy to go back home. However, we have been strongly in love for two years and three months but she then fell for another man, who didn't possess the girth of my penis. She had probably got used to it and needed another toy to play with.

Another of my gorgeous girlfriends was a married woman, again, with children, ten years older than me, again. Apparently, her husband has a very long and thick one and he can come and make her pregnant just like that. We connected on a deeper level though, not only beneath-the-belt level. Our souls embraced like Romeo and Juliet's. The matter was: 'Should I or shouldn't I'? She was an amazing entity in my life, the way she juggled between her work, family and myself. She is a risk-taker and she knew that our liaison could be dangerous as her husband seemed to be a very jealous and violent kind of guy. Even her siblings felt very concerned and kept on calling me to ask me to back off. We have seen each other a couple of times every year for the last three years. We were even planning a trip to Las Vegas to have loads of sex and play poker, so that I could escape my boring existence. But she realised I had no money and she didn't want to take that many risks with me.

When we were making love, it was like making a piece of art. Strokes were spontaneous and always perfectly expressed those blessed feelings of unity – unity of two in the boudoir and unity of oneself in the art studio. It is an exhilarating and liberating journey to attain the glory of a lady in a boudoir just like the glory of a piece of art is the completion of an internal picture's journey. Unfortunately, the beautiful inspiration she gave me won't happen again, as she has recently closed me off, preferring to respect the relationship with her husband. I feel sad, as I miss the beauty of her eyes and glorious body and our creative connection. But I am used to the rejection and I understand it anyway. This understanding helps me not to allow the pain to get me down.

My last girlfriend was training as a social worker and she madly fell in love with me during an art class. She was the same kind of woman as all my previous lovers: ten years older, married, frustrated with her sex and emotional life. And as usual I am an available escape option. She perfectly knew it was not ethical but she was totally overwhelmed by me. We met at my house many times. My family liked her, especially Matt, who always rejoices when I am happy. For a few months we met irregularly and talked on the phone until she decided to go to uni outside London. Off she went and I never heard from her again. I was sad for a few days and then went on with my life. I knew she wouldn't leave her husband for me, anyway, especially as he has a well-paid occupation.

Actually, this may be one of the major issues of my love life. Not being able to have a proper job and earn money is downgrading me at a deep level as it keeps women away from a long-term relationship. I have had a maximum of three jobs in my whole life, including a small role as an angel in an American thanksgiving movie called *Leprechaun*. I worked as a waiter for a luxury event organisation when I wasn't even 20. And then I worked seasonally as a landscape labourer for three weeks in my early twenties. I guess that we can't call any of these a proper job. I have enjoyed quite a few rich ladies for which money was not an issue but they were definitely not looking long term for a man who doesn't have a job. I realise that love is never unconditional, especially when money is involved, except for close family's love.

Truly one of my biggest regrets is not to be able to feel parenthood's unconditional love. Nevertheless, I am convinced that I will be a father one day, because I want to convince myself. Not being able to easily ejaculate in a woman's body is a sorry story for me as I would adore so much to become a father. However, I can still wank and come, although it doesn't give me an orgasm. So if a woman wanted to have a child with me it would not be difficult to wank and come inside her, as I have done many times in the past. Also, as my mother kindly suggests, I can put some sperm in the bank, waiting for Mrs Right. The real question is: Is there a lady around who can love me enough to deal with my disabilities and personality??? The women who floated my boat were all a bit bizarre, with other personality issues, and were mostly attracted by my looks, my super lovemaking and my disinhibited ways. This is the reason why I cannot mention all my amour-making stories, because some of these very sensitive ladies could take offence.

My super Tantric abilities have now left me and are only dependent on Viagra. I miss so much my immediate and long-lasting erections … I am told that lots of men go through the same disappointment after spending years fucking like rabbits. I understand that most young people can have sex for hours and then they move on to other priorities and more responsibilities. As I have no other priorities or responsibilities, keeping on fucking for hours was my favourite joy and also a way to escape my reality. Now I do miss making love a lot but at the same time I feel fine because I know I have had so much. I can afford a break, especially because my happy nature can afford it and my entourage is telling me it is better for my health. Writing this autobiography is helping me to discover a new self and a more balanced identity and I enjoy becoming more mature. Moreover, my sensuality and my tongue have not been damaged in any way by MS and my silver-tongued genius will probably be able to do its work on the pussy until the day I die.

Chapter 4

MS awareness

Viagra and a walking stick

My parents were extremely concerned with my future, making me aware of the development of the symptoms of MS and the need for a healthy lifestyle, but I was completely bored, annoyed and angry with their recommendations. Especially as I'd never had problems with my legs before the early years of 2000, I couldn't really understand that a healthy lifestyle was an absolute necessity. I should have listened to them – stupid of me!!!

I had lost the magic touch that I'd had on the football field in my schooldays for a few years but I'd managed to replace it with the ladies' touch in the boudoir. The erection problems arose together with the equilibrium problems. I started to lose my balance: sometimes I wouldn't be able to control my legs, sometimes they would feel heavy as lead, sometimes I was walking on broken glass, sometimes I was walking on ice, slipping around, and sometimes everything was fine. That is the effect that MS has on one's body. I needed a shoulder to lean on to walk or I had to grab things around me to steady myself. It felt like the ultimate punishment for having had such a skill on the football pitch.

I walked like I was drunk and it became impossible to get into clubs. I tried to tell bouncers that I had MS and wasn't drunk but couldn't help walking that way. It was before the Disability Discrimination Act and its rights were fully implemented. But they were only doing their job and just shooed me away. That was the beginning of my banning era from establishments. I didn't feel angry at them but it just added so much to my frustration not to be able to go out and have fun like any other young man. This was stopping me from meeting new ladies as well. Therefore, my neuropsychiatrist wrote a letter that I carried with me at all times confirming that I had MS and that it was affecting my balance. It did help.

Later, the reasons for my being banned changed. Fortunately, people were getting more aware of disability and how it can affect an individual but my social behaviour became more scary with the evolution of both MS and the bipolar condition. This double whammy made me very confused. I was becoming louder and louder and was stepping away from myself. I was high all the time, sometimes cool and sometimes irate. Anyway, at that time, quite fortunately, most pubs enjoyed welcoming drunk people. So I would come in swinging around, sober, and would ask for a triple CB. Indeed, Charlie Bacchus and Jack Daniels and Coke match well, even though I didn't need the Jack Daniels to open up, nor to get the girls attracted to me. I am naturally open, high and feeling free, even without any substance. It's just me on life. It adds to my good looks and is a great advantage I have to getting noticed. The girls wouldn't mind seeing me swinging around, because I'd tell them right away about the MS condition and that would bring sympathy.

It was certainly right after my first big heartbreak that my illness settled in and I started to use a walking stick. Until then the only symptom was a difficulty ejaculating, which taught me Tantric sex and made me a demi-god in bed. My heart was so broken, I felt like something vital had been taken away from me. My girly dream of marrying a princess had just gone, and my status as Prince had been crushed into gravel. I couldn't cry or express my pain in any way but my nerves suffered big-time and my illness came back in strength.

My swinging around took a dramatic step; grabbing things to keep my balance and support my 16 stones and heavy bones wasn't working anymore. I was falling down all the time. Fortunately, being a dribbler had taught me a good natural way of falling, as every opponent on the field would try to bring me down. Now I wasn't fighting to stand against the other team's defenders but was fighting just to stand up, against my own physical frailties and coping with the fact that my best skills were now my worst enemy. I never hurt myself falling down, but also because my nerves' illness avoided me feeling pain. The walking stick became essential and it felt like the ultimate grieving chapter – losing my legs, genius and my inner confidence.

At the same time, something bizarre happened to my erection. It stopped working so well. My dreams had already been destroyed when I knew I couldn't play football anymore. But taking away my sexual activity was even more cruel. It all started at that late, private, trendy, arty party. Garage music was banging, everyone was showing off their own style, trying to have fun. Standing out from the crowd, this beautiful gal was having genuine fun. Her sparkling personality touched me as much as her very big breasts. She knew how to handle those well (which I quickly learnt to do too). Not only did I love that about the woman, but I simply fell in love with her soul. Sally had such a strong and vibrant drive, always willing to go forward.

Unfortunately, when we arrived at her place later on that night, there was no more erection until the next morning.... That was the first time it had happened and then it became quite frequent. My Tantric sex nights, that helped me to cope with MS, were over. Although she was a bit younger than me, she was very strong with me, in mind, body and soul. Sally understood the situation and simply introduced me to Viagra. Before I had always told myself and others that I would never take Viagra. My pride and ego were really hurt, but it worked very well. Half a Viagra made me feel like a demi-god again and helped me to accept this new MS symptom.

We did do drugs together, and it changed Sally, who became detached from me (maybe she needed the drug to cope with my MS as well). However, we were both strong enough not to fall into any kind of addiction. I was very lucky to have her in my life at that time, supporting me going through that dramatic awakening of the MS awareness. We lasted three years. She came to live at my parents' house for some time. Everyone loved her, but it was not the most comfortable way to live and she finally had to move out. I was also happy to get my independence back.

Within three years, and that beautiful love, I changed from a sexy young man, acting without thinking much, into a walking-stick-and-Viagra-using man with a bit more depth than average. I was tired of sex gangsterism; it was now relationship time. Again, mania helped me cope and talk. When I should have felt depressed, I would just get naturally high to protect my soul and would add dope to it, which would take me much higher and help me forget. Also, Viagra would help my penis to get up and awaken the ladies.

It was impossible for me to accept that Viagra could further damage my nervous system because I did not want to accept that I had lost my demi-sex-god identity. The doctors checked my heart and thought it was so powerful, thanks to my sporting days, that I could deal with Viagra, so I kept on using it and got to taking four pills at once. The doctors told me that was very dangerous and can easily cause a heart attack. But one pill wouldn't be enough to last all night. It is quite impossible to leave that forcible place of a demi-god, satisfying the ladies in doing the ultimate sport, even if I know that ladies don't always enjoy long-lasting sex. It can hurt their sensitive pussy.

Anyway, I wouldn't wish this Viagra addiction on my worst enemy. I know it can kill but I feel I don't have much to lose. I also made money with it, selling 4 pills for 40 pounds, which got me weed. I managed to work it as a proper business, with several doctors involved. Of course, they didn't know how many I was using for myself and about the business made with them. My mum never knew about the business but later realised Viagra could be even more dangerous for me and simply took it away from me. I felt as if she had decided I should stop my sex life.

At times I felt exhausted for no apparent reason. This could last up to a week or even longer (I should say this fatigue is still here and is getting worse, even though I now use a wheelchair to go out and about). I used to glide, and now I was starting to feel my illness coming forth. My dream of playing football had passed away for ever. It had been with me for so long, even having been diagnosed with MS for several years, because I had no obvious symptoms and I was hanging on to a healing possibility.

Fortunately, too, my loving family was the best supporter and carer, even though being mothered and looked after all the time was (and still is) drastic. My parents had to curtail me in all my moves and that can be rather suffocating. The walking stick and the drugs were other kinds of supports supplied by the government but deep inside I often felt lost and I could hardly see a stream of fresh air to lift me up. However, the walking stick was definitely bringing some sympathy. As much as I don't like sympathy, it got me quite a few ladies, and it isn't as bad as pity.

Empathy, sympathy and pity

Pity is the worst that someone can show towards me. I know that it is a compassionate feeling but I don't like anyone feeling sorry for me. It infuriates me! I want to be able to play the cards that life has given me and certainly not be treated as a victim or a subhuman.

Some fine ladies can actually fall in love because they feel so sorry for me, whether or not they've had the Tantric sex experience. But then the relationship cannot be balanced enough: too much compassion keeps me in a restricted space and doesn't allow me to blossom and be in charge of my life. Too much sympathy also spearheads the pain, and this is also certainly bad for my damaged nervous system. It is interesting to note that the French word '*sympathie*' has got a much more positive meaning than 'sympathy' has in English. In French it goes with a happy smile and the will to share some good vibes; in English it is more of a feeling of condolence. I am still alive!!!

Empathy is a different caring emotion, where people are trying to get into my shoes and dare to ask questions and share back some feelings of understanding. They cannot share my own feelings, but at least expressing theirs towards me makes me feel respected and stronger inside. Somebody with pity would look at me with sad eyes and a frown but would hardly be able to smile frankly or talk to me; somebody with sympathy would try a bit too hard to be nice and comprehending when I don't need to be reminded every second how hurtful my situation is; whereas an empathetic person would not only give me a little smile but also give me a chance for a deeper connection and proper exchange.

Perhaps this is why I am trying to connect with every single soul I meet on the street. I obviously need to make sure people see me and recognise how active and happy I am from a wheelchair. I cannot help but talk loud to the world, because the world is a friend of mine. Loads don't even pay any attention to my greetings, which is quite normal, as they don't know me and consider me to be quite an alien ingredient in their life. I accept that, even if there may be sometimes some contempt in their attitude. Mostly, they don't want to be bothered and I respect that. Being ignored is not as bad as being pitied and reminded about the place I'm in. People with pity are nervous and try to get away quick. It hurts to feel that I am a thorn in their peaceful life.

However, 60 per cent of people *do* smile back, which is good enough for me; 50 per cent of that 60 per cent would talk back and a quarter of the people I talk to would engage in a proper conversation. So it is very much worth trying. This habit started after another heartbreak. I know it's such terrible behaviour; even my dad, who is the sweetest man on earth, doesn't want to go out with me. I am really interested in other people's lives as well, so we can share things. I especially enjoy talking to the ladies, as they can't help appreciating my outer beauty especially when I make them laugh, and they welcome me even more easily because I sound like a gentleman and look harmless. It's a fun game for me, because I know that I'm not that inoffensive. I love asking very private questions because it's a barrier breaker and it opens the doors to exciting times in the boudoir. I can't help telling everyone about my glorious adventures, even when some of them are just fantasies. This usually chases away any feeling of pity. Talking on the edge is my way to master the barriers provided by MS. It gives me the feeling that I am not the slave of that illness. I know this is a major symptom of my mania, which is quite helpful in my situation.

I can say that pity is the worst feeling towards me, as I have never felt aggression even though I know I can annoy people a lot sometimes and may deserve to be hushed up. I have the impression that even if they feel angry, they dare not have a go at me. And they definitely never show any hostility. There are many reasons for that. One of them is my disability, another one is my big smile and my fun take on life. When someone dares to give me a light frown, I just smile and go to the next table. Another reason may be that I don't feel any anger myself, so no one can catch onto that or take me up on it.

The only anger I can feel is the anger at myself when my disability holds me back, but usually I kind of accept that destiny with a smile and positive curiosity. I can get furious with my incapability to deal with my problems, especially when I've done or said something really stupid that has hurt someone I love – for instance, when I cheated on BIB with my sister's friend, or worse, when I get on the wrong side of my mum. Her pain hurts me beyond belief and even if I don't know why, I then know I have been pathetic. And she is still empathetic!

Serious people and experts keep on telling me that my fire dragon behaviour has accelerated my illness: never being careful with the cold or the heat, taking loads of drugs including Viagra, chain smoking, etc. I even have the feeling that shagging many women and not being serious enough to stick with one and build a family may have also hurt my nervous system. Being faithful and respectful to ladies and myself and keeping calm would probably have kept my nerves more controlled and content. My mania has helped me cope psychologically with the degradation of my body and my mental ability, but hiding the illness from my own self has not encouraged me to take care of those things.

I have been in denial of the seriousness of my illness. Both mania and my need to escape have prevented me from caring for myself properly but have also kept me alive and kicking. This is another reason why I hate pity, and even sympathy, so much, because they remind me of the situation I am so good at escaping from. I am glad I do not feel any pity for myself either; it would turn me into a drug addict. I have been relying on my mum as a nurse. Now that I am getting worse, I realise the gravity of the situation. Looking back on my life also helps me to accept the situation as it is and not cling to my previous escaping methods, such as gangster sex and drugs. I can see how strong the effect of drugs has been on my condition. But, of course, I just needed to fly away to a different land sometimes.

Oddly, writing this book is the opposite of escaping; it makes me embrace my situation. Strangely it does make me feel good to confront myself; it is helping me to find myself, to understand what has been going on in my life, in my body, my brain and my heart. I knew the whole story, but putting it into words makes it make sense. I can see the logic behind my behaviour and I can see the consequences too. It feels so good, remembering the good times, and also facing the bad times, as I sense I still own my whole life. I realise that memories are keys for the future. You can learn so much from them, what is good and bad, decent and indecent, the good things that have bad consequences. Whether they are positive or negative, they are friends who can guide you in your future. Actually, they are better than friends because you don't lose them.

Orally obsessed

Smoking the fag beyond the cut-off point, including the filter, burns both my fingers and my clothes. Effectively, when you reach the filter, the last burning bit is falling off. All my clothes are ruined.... It also burns my skin under my shirt without me feeling anything. My right index finger is so burnt my mother says it is going to fall off. I use a pumice stone to sand the stains and the burnt skin. I can sand it really hard without ever feeling anything. My neurological illness does not allow me to feel burning, cold, and all kind of physical reactions. This is the reason why I drop objects, because I don't feel them properly.... However, I do feel caresses, soft touches and hugs really well. And I love the stroke of the smoke in my mouth and in my respiratory system! It confuses me that I can't feel rough and extreme sensations; I can't always feel the things I am holding; sometimes I can't perceive the ground beneath my feet, but I'm always extremely sensitive to any gentle touch. How bizarre!!

Apart from catching the smoking habit from my adored grandparents, one of the reasons why I started smoking so heavily is because I had nothing left to lose – no sport activity requiring good health. Playing with my health has become a silly game. Why is it taking so long to take me away from this sorry existence? I know I will never commit suicide but ... I still need to drag the poison out of the cigarette as if I was looking for a lung cancer. It is a very sensual pleasure for my lips that may also be induced by the medication. I noticed that most people on heavy drugs, crack or neuroleptics, have that same smoking-the-life-out-of-the-cigarette compulsion.

Is there a link between drugs, cigarettes and quim licking? Is it relaxation starting in the mouth? Just like all kinds of positive emotions. If you love someone, you just want to talk or kiss her. Moreover, I love to lick out a woman, whether it's her pussy, her nipples or even her derrière. Am I obsessed? However, it seems that I discovered the glory of quim licking when I stopped having those undeniable erections lasting all night long....

I believe my first oral addiction was weed, not only loving its calming effects, but also the variety and subtlety of flavours. My favourite is sinsemilla because of its lovely rich taste and relaxing effects. Skunk is the most dangerous of all smokes. It is said that its THC rate is three times stronger but it does not calm at all; on the contrary it may awaken aggressive impulses. With me, as you know, there is no aggressiveness at all, but skunk can create a completely different person: I become agitated and loud and have a desire to lose my structured thought pattern. It can eventually make me feel happier for a short period but the after-effects are long and draining. Actually, the effects of skunk are the same as any other hard drug such as heroin, cocaine and crack: a quick high with long-lasting negative and heavy after-effects.

Sucking is another related part of my make-up which seems to be a regressive symptom that's developed since I started having difficulties fucking and not having so many girls to play around with. Especially when I'm resting, I automatically grab my necklace or a tissue or my shirt collar in my mouth. Like a baby, I need a dummy tit. I need to go back to that reliant state where you don't think, don't ask and just get loved. My tongue is still one of the most sensitive parts of my body, unlike the head of my penis, which has been one of the first parts of my body to lose sensation. Fucking and sucking are very close: they can both give great orgasms. Strangely, 'Fuck' and 'Suck' are also strong insults. How come things that can give so much pleasure are also an insult. They can also be complementary at least for me – the less I fuck, the more I need to suck. When I had a killer erection, I didn't need to go down at all. Now that I don't even fuck, I really need to keep on sucking something....

The licking impulsion is also a family tradition on my father's side. Licking plates like a dog bring us back to stone-age times and hasn't been cured by my education.

My tongue has acquired great skills in flexibility and sensitivity. However, I am not flexible enough myself and my dick is not long enough to allow myself to suck it, otherwise I would do it all the time. Would I, or wouldn't I? My tongue is also quite good at picking up tastes and is especially attracted by sweetness.

I have a very sweet tooth indeed. Unfortunately, I am not supposed to eat any sugar, for various reasons: sugar is not good for either my manic or my Candida conditions. When I eat too much sugar, I get excited, uplifted to a higher level. My mind takes everything in very quickly, just like when I was a child until I got sick. Back then I could focus very well and fast. Unfortunately, now my attention has become blunt and has a tendency to go all over the place. The focus seems to have disappeared. I know it's lurking somewhere. I also become even louder and more outrageous. At least that is the feedback I get from my peers when I talk to strangers in an open manner. It sounds rude to be interested in people's privacy. But I always am, and I love to talk to people. Is that another oral obsession?

The quim-licking obsession brought Candida onto my tongue, which consequently aggravated my addiction to sugar. Not many people know the strong links between the STD Candidiasis and sugar, as it usually sits in the sexual parts of the girl rather than in the man's mouth. It does make me crave for sugar, which further develops the yeasts. That consequence of my silver-tongue cavalier behaviour is definitely a very vicious circle, in all senses, good and bad.

Ahhhh! It leaves me with an infinite memory of my glorious sexual gangsterism.

I can also feel how fast my sugar cravings and addictions may put a whole load of weight upon me, quite heavy to carry. My stomach is the first one to grow, just like my Dad's and my bro's. I feel better and healthier with less sugar. When I make the effort, I am happy to fit into my chinos or my shorts and feel even sexier. Also, because it's becoming more and more difficult for me to climb the stairs, weight can be an issue.

I am happy to have the oral skill that gets the lady off. I am not ashamed it became an obsession with various oral symptoms; some of them could kill me but they do give a good taste to my existence on this glorious planet.

Positivity between a rock and a hard place

This is how I've been feeling for many years. The rock is me getting MS at 17 and the hard place is the life that I have to live. Mum was the main cushion between the rock and the hard place, and still is. Girlfriends and friends are also there to cuddle my spirits. Matt is more than the biggest cushion; he is both a pillow and a warm blanket. He naturally knows how to escape his own hard rock and place by just living in the moment, here and now. I learnt that key to happiness from him, just being with him, feeling graciously lively and connected to each other and to the cosmos.

Life with MS is a mess, and being MSsy is getting very tricky at times. As my brother shows me, the best way to deal with it is to seize the day, to feel alive – I felt so alive when I played football. But this MS is a good trick God is playing on me; it's got me deeper than you can even imagine, physically with my tongue and my dick, and mentally as well. It's also got me higher, to another plane; art and dope go together very well for creation's sake.

I have been athletic since birth, kicking very much in the womb (I even like to think I had a six-pack at birth) so getting MS was the worst thing that could ever happen to me, as it does have a cut-off point. Football will always be within my soul. Even though my memory is leaving me, I still have vivid images and feelings of the games, and especially the impact I had on the game when I had my striker boots on. I miss it so much; I cannot tell you. When I think about it or when I see a match on TV, I have a very strange mixed feeling of deep sorrow and pride. I am very used to that ambivalent feeling within. I miss the fact that I should be on TV as well. All this has been stolen away from my existence but not from my soul. Even though life has robbed me off my sporting days, I know that a champion does not last for ever and I am still very confident about my bright future. My confidence has definitely supported me in this drastic life change. Even better: the more my body transitioned into a man using a wheelchair, the more my spirit grew and strengthened. The low points are there but they never ever last more than a few minutes.

In attacking my frontal lobe, MS forced my brain to open up and get out of its trap. I was and still am drawn to people – especially happy ones, needing to share love and find recognition of my existence. It's not only the ladies but the entire world that I want to love and that I'm interested in. This is the reason why I developed this unique habit of talking to every single person I meet on the street, not only because I need to be seen and heard (I easily tell them about my life when they just dare to look at me) but also because I need to share, and I am genuinely interested in other lives and am always looking for love. That aspect of my bipolarity is a gift allowing me an exciting existence and keeping me positive, spiritual and fulfilled.

This bizarre habit attracts all kinds of people – many of the lost ones who can find in me a new potential friend, or victim. Indeed, the most vulnerable people turn to me like straw to water, especially those like me who need an audience and have a lot to say but are rarely listened to. I am happy to listen to them and discover their interesting journeys. This is how I make so many 'friends/girlfriends'. They make me realise how lucky I am to be born into my family. My area used to be my lair. First, I used to play football there. Then I would meet there so many fascinating people, who would be trying to escape the world just like me but in a very different manner. Being a vulnerable person myself, I relate to vulnerable people very well. It seems that helpless people are also attracted by me. I cannot run away, stuck to a stick or a chair, and my strong spirits and ever-smiling face never dismiss them. We shared the love for weed or cigarettes and a few drinks as well.

I am glad I didn't fall into alcohol as much as I fell into weed, probably because of my education. Those wasters knew how to retain whatever was in my pockets and wallet. I have rarely been to the place they lived in, only through curiosity, or God only knows what may well have happened. Indeed, curiosity may have killed the cat but I know my limits very well, even though my parents believe I don't. I have never ever slept with any girls hanging around on the Common. Even if I fancied a few, I just knew it wouldn't be right to go that way, whether it is my instinct or my education.

It was strange to hang around with the lost souls in the very same place where I was attaining my best skills in life. Also weird to find so much entertainment with these people. We had such good laughs, free to be as delirious as ever, with no judgement; living life on the edge, we were the injured souls of the Common blessed by Florence Nightingale's statue and spirit. It is also a great opportunity to learn about various professional activities or other subjects that can obsess people. I had a nice course on natural diets and herbs. I got to know the most amazing transvestite. I was happy to meet guys who would share my same female obsession. Moreover, the strong feeling of solidarity gave each of us some worth and respect. We were in the same sinking boat with mental health issues but all with strong spirits, able to keep a smiley face above the water, recognising and helping each other, and keeping on laughing despite the misery of our lives.

In 2004, even though I was using a stick, I was feeling so well balanced mentally, thanks to good medication and a joyful sex life, that my mum tried to further my life, using my knowledge of disability and my love for art and business. She found this great opportunity to work as a disability trainer in an organisation promoting arts and business. I managed to go through the first interview on a breeze because I had put together – with the help of Mum of course – an efficient portfolio presenting myself and my artwork. One of the interviewers was too cute and sexy for words. Our unconscious flirting during the interview probably helped with my enrolment. I was given a lesson plan with good resources that I had to explain to ten disabled trainees. Unfortunately, that same beautiful sexy lady was one of the observers of the session. She not only observed but also smiled in an engaging manner. She reminded me of an ex-lover and this drove my mind away from the course. The only thing I can remember now is how the powerful feeling of having an audience, including a fanciful lady, helped my mind to escape into my favourite subject and I became a comedy-club star addressing an oration about my beautiful sexual life. Maybe I realised it would be more fun and useful to teach about sex than business. Of course, that was not the intention of my mother. So my career as a trainer died a sorry, funny death. However, that sexy lady and I had exchanged numbers and we had fun on a later date....

Now the use of a cheap wheelchair doesn't allow me to escape, neither to the realms of lonely princesses nor to the land of the lost souls anymore. I suspect my parents find it safer for me not to be able to have a proper wheelchair that I could handle all by myself. I may scoot away.

Dreaming to leave the family home

The drug and sex bingeing went on for about 16 years and the drug attraction is still there as a quick escape from my condition. Even though my parents were not totally aware of all my outbreaks, it was difficult for them to cope with and they had to put down some boundaries so that it didn't invade their life too much. My mum had to control me as if I was a young teenager. At some point, I felt that she was willing to stop my sex life by controlling my use of Viagra, which I understand now was really too much. She has taken my mobile phone away a few times to make sure I don't call dodgy people to the house or stray for drugs or to keep me away from a troubled lady who was hassling me.

This woman, my mother, got so much on my nerves that I had to torch my shorts to show my fury in a moment of defiance and defence. Of course, it was a very childish thing to do but the only way for me to put up with an over-controlled life and again challenge my freedom. It is such a vicious circle as it forces Mum to be willing to control every single move I make and all my links to the outside world. She has also kept my ComCab card, my wallet and my cashcard. She did that after my last drugs extortion on a night when she and my father went out to the theatre. This is a vicious circle because the more I'm locked in, the more I wish to escape, even if I completely understand that she is doing all this to protect me from myself and from being exploited. It is disturbing, as I understand her points, but possession is nine-tenths of the law.

Treating me like a kid is not going to help me grow, even though she has good reasons for not trusting me at all. Actually, both my parents have not trusted me since my sex gangsterism period and drug addiction. As a finale, I feel this is a double bind because I love Mum so much and I know I can be a danger to myself, but her restraint only leads me to more craziness if I haven't been able to discuss, think and write about it. It is true that I have been barking down the wrong alley for quite a number of years in my life. So now I understand Mum's reasoning for trying to limit my chances of escape to other worlds that are especially dangerous for my condition. Not being able anymore to read and write, nor walk or run, I can just watch TV and wait for my personal assistants (PAs).

My parents know that without any freedom or independence, I will stray. Therefore, I definitely need to take a step to prove to them that I need more independence and respect to feel my life has some purpose. I know I need to show my maturity and respect to them, and talk to them about it. But for some reason it is very difficult for me to do so. Being treated like a child but not being a teenager anymore, it is extremely difficult to address freely my issues and negative feelings. It is easy to do so with my French psychologist-PA who is digging into my soul to write this book, but it seems so hard to do it with my mother. I love her so much and am so dependent on her power, it is eating away at me. Or am I still in my Oedipus complex, in love with her and not able to grow apart.

Maybe I should reaffirm to my parents how much I understand that drugs have had a negative effect on my neurological system, how much my crazy behaviour must have hurt them. I should talk seriously about future plans and refrain from talking about my previous crazy sex-life or my fantasies all the time. I need to manipulate them harder than ever, because they know me so well.

A TV channel asked to interview me for a programme on disability. Because my mum was controlling my phone, she got their request and decided this would not happen unless she could control it. It is getting worse, because now she wants to shackle my thoughts as well, always with a protective goal, protecting me from being exploited. She thinks that the TV interviewer is going to take advantage of me and put me in bad light, and that could make me lose my benefits. I know that the British media can do anything, including spending loads of money to take over a story and make it sound sensational against the person's privacy and/or reality. The simple truth is not as important to them as the opportunity to create a scoop and make money. People's respect is their last consideration. They know how to exploit the general public's natural curiosity for filth, violence and insanity. Disability is also something that can fascinate people, because they are fearful and happy to have escaped from it. My life is quite insane as well. However, I would have really enjoyed showing off on TV and talking about all my adventures, especially with the ladies.

Although we love each other so much, both my parents and I are often really fed up to be living together. Finding my own accommodation is always an urgent and hot issue. My mum fights like a howling wolf for her puppy to get me a decent future, but nobody is listening. Because of bipolar and MS, none of those caring bodies would take responsibility but instead were happy to get rid of me by bouncing me back and forth between social services, the neurological department and mental health services, without addressing jointly my two conditions. They were prompt to argue that my bipolar condition is not dangerous for other people and that I am very fortunate with my white middle-class family and its big house in a catchment area. We cannot judge people by their wealth/colour/class, but it is true that I am luckier than most.

Though obviously interested in my needs for independence and my happy disposition, smiley face and dynamic blue eyes no one would help to convince them. I felt like a lost diamond in the rough. My mother fought so much that we finally got in a health professional, an amazing commissioner for adult services at the health authority. This lady certainly opened our eyes to my condition. She spent hours talking with me and trying to understand me, which I appreciated more than ever, especially as she had the right medical knowledge and experience. She had seen many patients with complex behaviour who had MS. Her view was that my difficulty with boundaries was due to MS rather than bipolar, because of the frontal lobe damage. Therefore, I was back into the hands of the health services. In order to get proper residential housing with 24-hour support, I needed to go to this transitional rehabilitation centre first, which was supposed to be the last official step before moving away from the family household.

I was so happy with that prospect that I agreed right away. And off I went to a renowned neurological rehabilitation centre in November 2011. It appeared that the longer I stayed there the better care and freedom I might get out of it. But if I'd known I'd be stuck there for five months – without any sex and only weekends for family love – I would probably have refused to go, thinking it may have driven me much more insane than I was.

I had my own bedroom, basic hospital style, where I brought in my own TV, but could only have very few visitors there.... It was impossible to go out without an officially 'reliable' friend or member of the family. It was like a hotel with rules. The staff were beautiful, looking after me, always available and checking all my needs (except the sexual ones, which drove me crazy). I regularly met with a psychologist to discuss how I was feeling. He was very helpful. He was so touched by the piece of art I gave him that he hung it in his office. A middle-aged nurse from South Africa understood me particularly well, especially as I had to face MS getting far worse. I got introduced to a wheelchair – which I used most of the time – and started to settle into the status of a disabled man. Everyone in the family sent me beautiful cards and my favourite pieces of artwork were on the walls. I went back home every weekend, where I also felt locked in.

Strangely it took me two months to find out I could register for the art club. My 'inmates' and I were spending most of the time smoking cigarettes in the garden or watching TV. The only official occupation was daily discussion groups ran by nurses (they were all beautiful and sweet) around the daily news in the papers. The exercise was to rewrite headlines after reading a chosen article. Unfortunately, I could not read properly – because of MS – so I would only get a few words from the article and elaborate from the original headline. I really enjoyed those morning sessions because everyone was interested in what I had to say. I was obviously the most alive person in the group of patients, happy to express my opinions and feelings. It seemed I was taking over, as I could be told off by some patients. Other inmates had various kinds of neurologic ailments, all dealing with life kicking the thrust within. Many conversations took place outside the morning discussion groups. My mother says that everyone loved me.

I am aware that these five months away brought some rest to me and the family. I do miss it sometimes, this feeling of fraternity where we all share some heavy loads and can support each other. I keep looking at a picture of me and my closest mates in the centre. It was quite a meeting of minds. H is an Italian masterful one, whose Christianity was so powerful that it got in the way of his mental agility. M is a Moroccan guy who used to be a drug dealer and his new-found faith gave him the mental balance he needed. God's ways are definitely mysterious. He is up in heaven having a laugh at the impact of his universal love.

Happy to be away from the family pressure and allowed to be myself, even though it was in a very restrained environment, I felt I was in a friendly prison. Of course, I tried to flirt and joke with the nurses, knowing they were too professional to let me and my tongue in(side). Therefore, the only oral satisfactions left were fags, sweets and lollipops. I was so bored that I kept on eating sweets and put on quite a lot of weight – the addiction due to the Candida in my mouth had not been discovered yet but the symptoms were there!

However, these five months of assessment didn't even manage to achieve the goal to find me a home outside the family. There are too many people needing care with less fortunate family situations. The fight for independence has been going on since, even though it means 24-hour care and spying on me. What a paradox! I like to think my life is a fun game to play. At some point I was found a flat to share with other individuals but it was up north and we all agreed that it was too far for the family to visit. My hero Matt and myself would have missed each other too much. I know that living in a care home will make me even more dependent on people who won't be as loving, available and patient as my family. However, I am ready to make that step to try to get independence from the family and especially from my mum and ultimately to have a chance to live my own life and grow up a bit.

My mother is such a great mum but she is getting older, tired and more anxious about all of us. Maybe this is why I have the impression that she may become more and more controlling. She deserves a proper retirement. These are other good reasons why I want to get out of this house. I still want to believe that I will feel more independent when I leave. Even though it would be less comfortable, I would love to get away from here, to have a true existence and to feel who I really am. I want to be true to myself. Unfortunately, I have the impression that my Mum's love, care, power and attentiveness do not allow me to be myself. I even find it very hard to express myself to her. I feel like I am still a baby when I am just discovering that I can live without my drugs and sexual urges – another paradox of my existence. It may be harder to live in a care home, but I need a change and I need to see who I am in society, how I'll cope with my dependencies. I want to become far more responsible and need to find a new self, a beautifully balanced 'CB'. I like to think that the time and place I'm in is very comfortable, just because of my pleasure-seeking mind that helps tone things down. I know at times I can deny reality. I am no longer the beautiful sportsman I used to be. But I am still feeling very happy within myself, and this is probably the most important thing in life.

The ideal situation would be to have a woman who is paid to take care of me and we would unite in a positive relationship. It is worth taking the risk to get out of here.

A final solution has been found to fit with the social services care plan, my physical condition and the fact that Mum is getting older: my parents have organised the double sitting rooms downstairs as my own apartment. The front room will be my bedroom and sitting room. I will have my own bathroom built. There will be a door out to the garden for me to go out and smoke. There will be a mini kitchen with my microwave and fridge, which will give me more independence. And I will be even more in the middle of the family life, between the front door and the kitchen. My parents are now organising the first floor to become their sitting room and Matt will take up my old room on the top floor in the roof. It will also be easier for my PAs to be here with me without intruding on the family life too much.

This is a very difficult step for me to take because I don't feel it is my own decision, even though I was consulted. I realise that my main issue is leaving behind all my visual memories of my twenties and of being on both my legs: all those romantic, mischievous and sometimes very hot activities in the attic room I grew up in. I was the prince of that lovely boudoir, under the stars. And now the only plan is to regress downstairs. It is true that the most important thing is to care for my safety, as my balance is getting worse. But getting worse is never in my mind; I never think that way and will never do. I trust other people to do that for me.

The main issue is that Mum is not strong enough to hold me up anymore. However, I know I can keep the best memories intact and very much alive in my brain, especially when I am on good form. Since I'm not going on binges I'm on even greater form. That new room could be a new studio and a new start in a new life. I will be happy to have all my best artwork framed and hanging. I will also get rid of many of my childhood and adolescence memories although I will definitely keep my sport trophies. I guess that a decluttering of 15 years will be *very* refreshing. My actual attic room is a big mess with a lot of family junk. I have felt like Tarzan in the jungle attracting a mate. Now I want to be a gentleman in a clean and fresh environment. It will be a great change, like going on holiday. This will allow a new PA to come and stay with me most of the time to give Mum and my family a break.

Also, I love the idea that Matt will really enjoy living in this attic room and I can visit him in my ex-room. The only thing that I will really miss is to follow the ladies' derrières upstairs. It is interesting to see how writing this has helped me to accept this change. I am now able to talk about it with the family and project myself in my own new space. I will be able to invite friends and do my own things without begging anyone. It is quite incredible how my opinion has changed after going through the regret. Because I was so sad about leaving some of my best times memories and perturbed at not being involved in the initial decision, I just wouldn't even think about it. As a matter of fact, this is my way of reacting to negative thoughts – to just cancel them out from my consciousness. This self-protection usually helps a lot, but it really doesn't help to clear the problems out. Now I know that I can miss this room and its memories as one part of my journey that is over. Decluttering makes me feel good, as it makes me feel more in control of the present and aware of building a new future.

Falling into a wheelchair

It drove me crazy, after my sporting history: being in a wheelchair forces me to accept my condition and my vulnerability. Feeling people's respect and care helps this acceptance. I can see love in their eyes. It makes me feel ambivalent again … Feeling lucky about my parents and all the love and intelligence around me and at the same time feeling the illness taking over my whole life. Being a child forever in my parent's home and being bored at the age of 36.

I am six foot two, handling the world from a few feet below when I am out and about on this wheelchair, just like a baby in a pram. Besides, it's quite bizarre when I pass a baby in a pram looking directly at me puzzled how huge and beardy this big baby is. It takes me directly back to my own childhood. Actually, me being in a wheelchair is like being in a spaceship without any fuel.

I don't like to be pushed around, but it's not an easy thing for me to handle my wheelchair on my own; it seems that I'd rather be pushed than be self-reliant. I find all kinds of reasons not to manoeuvre the wheelchair myself. Is it safety first? That's not true, because I always like to take risks, even if that worries my parents. The reason is probably that I cannot trust myself physically nor mentally. It is difficult for me to accept another lack of self-control, especially with the tool that could give me some freedom. It is difficult for people to believe me when I justify my laziness, saying that I'm not strong enough or that the chair isn't good enough or that I'm giving people the opportunity to show what they're good at. Maybe the main reason for my laziness about pushing myself around is the satisfaction of ordering people around and getting some power from being useless and in a 'pram'. Also, it's a confusing feeling of being in front and ordering people around but never being sure of which way they're going to go – if they're going to miss that step and make me feel totally out of control.

I do enjoy being pushed. I need to be pushed physically and mentally as well. Do I enjoy regressing in various fashions? It's a very bizarre feeling to be pushed by my mum especially; I love and hate it all at once. It's like Thanks and Piss Off, I hate U MS!

Actually, my relationship with the wheelchair completely depends on the power I feel within. If I'm feeling bad, whether it's mental or physical, I'm unable to spin those wheels. It took me about 18 months to get used to the chair and that disabled status. Now I realise how much freedom it can bring me; I do dare to push myself more. I am even thinking of becoming a wheelchair champion. But I don't know where to start and I feel too lazy to practice. I am afraid I have got addicted to laziness as a side-effect of MS.

Nevertheless, the need of a wheelchair makes me an official disabled person, which means I can have support from carers/personal assistants up to 25 hours a week, which is changing my life and my mum's life as well. It also makes me eligible for my own accommodation, which may never happen.

My personal assistants

Falling into a wheelchair allowed me to have first 12, then 18 hours and now 24 hours of assistance a week. I am helped by a service called Direct Payments which was campaigned for by disabled people. Fortunately, the Direct Payments procedure allows us to choose the personal assistants I want.

The PAs are completely changing mine and my mother's life, even though it is a lot of HR and admin work for Mum. I feel very relaxed with my PAs; I feel a deep love for them because they are there for me 100 per cent; they have no pity, but enough compassion to understand where I am coming from. They are quite patient, and it is good for them to be impatient sometimes, to put me back in my place and to express their frustration. They are all very intelligent people. Both my Mum and myself prepare interviews well, with quite deep questions. More importantly, we are both lucky to be able to feel people's souls, especially when they are transparent, loyal and fun-loving like us. We were very lucky with the people we found. Each one has the right calibre for their specific task. We did employ a trainee doctor just in case one of the PAs couldn't make it. But they are all present, on time, smiley and energetic. They say that working with me gives them energy and makes them smile. They also say that they feel very free to be themselves because I am a free spirit. We can agree to disagree and have arguments. I feel that arguments always resolve the case, avoiding cynicism and bitterness. Even better, a dispute can raise deep communication and help us understand each other much better, and we then become closer friends.

Also, my PAs enjoy the fact that I am always happy and moreover never angry. I can be sad or confused but never resentful nor aggrieved. The only things I can be angry about are war or injustice or bad treatment of children. I do feel sorry for myself at times. Fortunately, my PAs often encourage a fun mood or just a different mood or perspective. They also bring some fresh air from outside, and even sometimes they can bring me some new friends. I can be myself 100 per cent and I feel very comfortable with them. I like their empathy, as they also feel comfortable to talk about anything and express their feelings about my situation. Their professional status protects them from falling into the trap of emotions or a dependency/power relationship. It also helps them to set boundaries. For instance, a friend would feel bad about telling me off. My PAs and I are kindred spirits. It is very interesting and positive to see how those professional boundaries also allow us to feel close and comfortable, just like a family or a squad. The good thing is that we don't see each other too much.

In the past, I was always trying to escape from my condition with ladies or drugs. Now I am alive with my own personal activities. Being able to have physical, mental, creative and entertaining activities mostly outside home, makes me feel sprightly and complete.

JF, the young medical student, was the first employed PA and he helped me out at Bable. Bable was a free play that I was part of that was performed outside in a park, which was something my mum helped me be part of. This is where I started telling my story and which led me to want to continue on with writing. JF also took me to the gym once a week for hydrotherapy, which keeps my muscles strong and active. He also took me to my medical appointments. I get on very well with him. It's good to have a male friend to talk to about women and life. He is a cool guy who manages to get away on holiday on a regular basis. Therefore, JF helped to find another medical student as a PA to replace him when he wasn't available. Because of his studies, he couldn't carry on working with me. However, we have stayed good friends and I do miss him sometimes. I was really really touched in my deep heart to be invited to his wedding. It was an amazing party where I kept my whole table laughing and met a few incredible people.

> I met Charlie four years ago through his cousin Ralph who is a friend of mine from the University of Leeds. Ralph told me about the newly created PA hours Hannah, Charlie's mum, had fought to get. I needed a job and was training to be a doctor so it seemed like a good idea. It may work out particularly well for me as Charlie has promised that when he makes his millions, he'll employ me to work privately in Barbados. My fingers are still crossed. I'll admit that the first few times we met were tough. Both physically and socially demanding. I was nervous about what I should and shouldn't do and, as Charlie knows, well he can veer to the side of socially unacceptable when given the opportunity. But over time we developed a fantastic rapport and I soon got over my initial lack of confidence. The first times I worked with Charlie was also an acting job as Charlie was working on a community theatre production called Bable. Charlie thrives in such an environment and his natural charm shines through. After Bable with Charlie we spent a large amount of time frequenting cafes that by complete coincidence had attractive young women working in them. Also by complete coincidence we often tried new places if we'd been served by men. His natural charm makes him an instantly likeable character. Charlie often refers to himself as the 'Silver-Tongued Cavalier', and when in public this is an apt way of describing him. I am yet

to meet someone who didn't find him charming. A small criticism might be that he can sometimes be a little too charming! I enjoyed our bus journeys during which Charlie says hello to every passenger. In modern London having a conversation with a stranger on a bus is a rarity, but with everyone must be pretty much unheard of unless you know Charlie. Working with Charlie helped me to develop professionally, but much more importantly it gave me the opportunity to make a new and important friend.

Four years after I met Charlie and we are still close. Although I am busy with studying in central London a lot of the time so we don't meet up as often as I'd like. Nowadays I meet up with Charlie without the guise of employment. We've been able to get to know each other in a new light. I enjoy going to his birthdays and when we meet up for lunch or a coffee. His family is very important to him and I greatly enjoy seeing Hannah, Rob and Matt whenever I have the opportunity to. There is a closeness and supportiveness in their family, with each member playing an important role, that I admire and hope to emulate in the future myself.

Charlie has taught me a huge about the human condition and I will be eternally grateful to him for letting me be a part of his life in the past and in the future.

JF

JF also replaced A who used to take me to the gym. A is a lovely young nurse who used to take me to the cinema every week; good job for her, she was paid to go to the cinema with free tickets. Her main job was to help me find a seat and take me to the toilets in the middle of the film. I know it is not an easy task anyway. We would usually have a coffee afterwards. She is one of the rare people who never minded my oversocial ways, and deserves an award for that. She is so cool; she brought her best friends to my party and that rocked. Unfortunately for me and good for her, she got a proper job nursing.

Another young beautiful PA, V, was employed to take me both to art lessons at the art centre and to cycling sessions once a week. She also helped me with my shopping and cooking. We had really great conversations about everything and anything, sometimes deep and always interesting. She is such a beautiful sexy and warm South American girl that I could not help fancying her. I had to learn to control my desire for her, with her help. Maybe because of this frustration, I sometimes behaved badly when around her. Once I remember V got very angry and disgusted. We were in a café and I started licking the table where I'd spilled custard, which meant that I also had custard all over my face. I can remember her expression of disgust which still hurts me when I think about it. It made me realise what I had just done; I was a fool and felt shocked about my own disgusting behavior. To relax a bit, I lit a cigarette but that was just too much for V, who couldn't stand me smoking inside and decided to leave the coffeeshop immediately.

I don't care about looking stupid in public. But I feel really bad when I offend and disgust a beautiful lady and a good friend. Another time we were in the bus going back from the art school with a delicious pavlova that I had asked Mum to cook for my art colleagues for Christmas. Unfortunately, they were too busy to even taste it because they all wanted to finish their art-work for Christmas. So I was left with my pavlova and ate it in the cab in my disgusting, worse-than-animal-like fashion, both hands into it and filling my mouth like a starving slave, plus throwing pieces at V's face and all over the cab. I always wonder why I behave in such stupid fashion and how I can learn how to repress myself. I still feel I was an idiot, big time! I know it is my frontal lobe that is a bit damaged.

Anyway, V got angry and took some time off. It hurt my feelings a lot to lose her because of my stupid behavior. Mum and V had a really good conversation and we managed to get her back. One of the most amazing and touching things she did was a collage picture as a present for my thirty-fifth birthday. Not only beautiful and creative, this picture manages to be very realistic and abstract at once! People say that she really got my true personality and reality shining through. It also reminds me of my days playing football on the Common. She left me again for a proper job in a Latin American charity and a film course. Good for her! And may be good for me as she is thinking about doing a video about my daily life. We are still catching up once in a while as friends. I will always love you V!

Something we need to discuss, even though I am not really proud of it, is how I try to empower myself with every new PA. I use their politeness and willingness to satisfy me to impose my will and sometimes do silly-billy things that my family and my other PAs would not accept. I can push the boundaries with new PAs until they feel so uncomfortable about it that they talk to my mum. It is my way of escaping my condition. And my PAs quickly understand that, but also learn to help me. It is not too difficult for them, as I am stuck in that wheelchair.

My most tip-top PA is the lady who helps me write this book you are reading. Mab is like my ultimate big sister. As with my dearest grandma, I can tell her everything in the world and she will keep the secret, unless I decide to disclose it in this book. It may come up in a following book. Mab and I are working on bringing out my most exciting stories, inner feelings and thoughts – some of them have never been put into words before, giving them a boundary to run up against. So many people have so many thoughts that they hide away from themselves. As a trained psychologist she enjoys digging up things, words and feelings out of my brain and helps wind them up and clarify my own dark clouds. I enjoy it a lot because it is a platform to play upon and gives sense to my life. Sometimes we argue, because she is fed up to be the one digging into my brain and looking for the right words about my own existence, especially as she is French and suffers from lack of vocabulary. She is keen to learn though. Nevertheless, she finds me quite lazy. She doesn't know if it's due to my condition or if I just enjoy having a lady taking care of my good and bad self and waiting for her to make me feel like the masterful one.

When I fall asleep for a few minutes, she can also rest upon her chest and better concentrate on the book. Thanks to her Latin roots, she is very free-minded and has fun talking about sex. Discussing my most favourite subject with no limits makes me the happiest man in the world. It is great to have a female point of view and get both sides of the coin. She insists that most young men can fuck for hours and I was not that exceptional. She wouldn't agree to talk about her own sex life though. I don't mind when she brings me back down to earth, it makes me feel more human. Actually, I am always so proud to have been through this amazing journey as a simple human. I felt I was an angel already back there when I was flying around the pitch, playing football when I was young. I felt like an angel when I was a real catch for the ladies.

And I still enjoy feeling like an angel to escape my reality. My weakened frontal lobe makes me believe in my dreams very strongly. For instance, I am convincing myself that I'm going to play football again, become very rich with this book and get so many ladies people won't believe. 'Of course they won't!' says Mab with a twist and a chuckle. I will deny her until she manages to convince me. It is really strange how my brain often works in a different manner to reality and agrees to come back to life without feeling irritated. Mab is bringing me back to reality in a cooler manner than my family, because she doesn't have to stand against my good self all day long. Mab and I have had so many intimate conversations and shared so much that I feel like we could build something together and I asked her to marry me a few times, but she has denied me. She has got enough with these few hours a week. And this book is our baby. It doesn't wake us up at night. She is such a beautiful lady that I love her big-time. She gave my journey a fantastic new direction, understanding myself more deeply.

R is the best PA I could ever have. He is a handsome young man of 23 and studies physiotherapy. He started as my physiotherapist, taking me to the gym every week and sometimes making me work out in my bedroom. As I haven't had any other kind of physical exercise in my boudoir for quite a while, it is helpful to still use it to tone my muscles and drill my whole body. R is impressed with my very muscular body. Years of intensive football have left me with a lot of frustration but also with a great body, which is quite helpful right now. It is also my genes that gave me that great body and the illness as well.

When R and I are on the street, we both enjoy attention from the ladies. R understands where I am coming from, especially as we often talk about girls together. He is fun and wise as well. He is so serious that he prefers to focus on his work right now rather than spend time and money on girls. He doesn't mind too much me talking to everyone around. He just sometimes asks me to shut up, like everyone else does. He is so focussed on everything he is doing; what a professional young man! He is so dedicated that I accept easily when he is a bit over-protective and controlling of me. I kind of like being controlled by a cool dude like him. It makes me feel secure, as I do feel he always acts for my best interests as a real friend and a very responsible PA. He went with us on holiday to Spain where we went swimming quite a lot. It feels like he is part of the family. He is gregarious like us. I feel he is like a brother and I wish him luck for the future as I know he is very intelligent. I would like him to stay with me as we have very strong respect for one another. Good luck, R!

> Charlie Bacchus, the man to be, the silver-tongued cavalier, the man with two faces and the Scorpio fire dragon. These are all names that I and the local people – possibly the whole of CB's area of town it feels at times – have heard when meeting this gentleman.
>
> I should rephrase that last word, gentleman. Perhaps it should read: gentle man. To me he is simply 'C' and less simply, he has grown to be more than a job, more than a nine to five. He has become my friend, my ally and to be bloody honest, it feels like more of a brother relationship. I say this because of how we act and react to each other during our time together. The way we can have a snappy argument about him wanting to swindle that one extra cigarette, do one less exercise at the gym or pool or whether it is shouting across the road to a rather lovely looking lady. Until one minute later when he is asking about how my mum or brother are doing – remembering facts that I have forgotten, about their jobs or lives that I have spoken to him about. I say gentle man because this is what he is; a kind-natured, loving man who holds his family and friends in the highest regard.

Perspective – 18 months ago when C and the Matriarch interviewed me to come on board, we spoke a lot about what I could offer him, the good I could do to enrich his life, support him. Not once did we speak about what C could offer me. I have never known someone who wants to speak to every single person passing by. Even at a crossing when a car pulls up with the window open! – 'Hello good sir' he will shout, even if it is a woman. You can't help but laugh. Live, love, laugh. The resolve this man has shown when faced with multiple sclerosis is inspiring. C has had MS for nearly the summation of my entire life.

Perspective – he loves, he laughs and he lives. This man has my respect and my love. He isn't a job, he is my friend and it truly is a pleasure coming to see him weekly and being able to impact his life in the same way that he impacts mine.

There is so much I can say about this man, anecdotes both funny and sad. But to you, Charlie, I leave you with this. No matter where I am, what I am doing – I will carry a part of you with me. You have grown to be one of my best friends, hell – we even spent Easter together playing board games! I wish you all the best with this novella, and I cannot wait to finally get my hands on a copy to truly know everything about the silver-tongued cavalier. Carpe Diem my friend, Carpe Diem.

All my love,
Robin

Writing the book in my own bedroom is especially fulfilling. I feel like a convalescent, as I am stepping away from invading emotions and obsessions in looking at them. It is not only fun to share my adventures; it is momentous to write down all these incredible events that built myself as I am today. It seems to me that now it all make sense. Reviewing and connecting all the events of my life gives me another perspective on everything. Mab says I am doing the brain job of a teenager: developing my frontal lobe that has been fucked up by MS to differentiate and connect my various thoughts, knowledge and emotions. This is hopefully strengthening my thinking and will reduce my impulsivity! We are not there yet. However, reflecting on my own self makes things more interesting and deeper. My journey has been so incredible.

About freedom, clairvoyance and vulnerability

It was a great coincidence that my birthday party happened on Halloween night. We did it at a pub where they had organised a proper Halloween party with dead people and scabs hanging outside, a décor of mist, an excellent DJ and a bunch of amazing devils, dead people and witches with extraordinary costumes. Everyone was smiling and willing to have fun. Actually, there was a big banner saying 'This is Halloween night, if you don't want to party, fuck off!!'. I had been hassling everyone about this party for months. Each year on my birthday I do my best to celebrate myself. I believe that if you have had a good year it will show in the party.

Unfortunately, my previous parties didn't happen really well. People would not show up, I would get really pissed and bored, and nothing interesting would happen. But this year was all different. I had sent a text invite to officialise the event. I was lucky to have my four PAs around, bringing their friends and lovers, cakes and wine. My mum baked my favourite extra-large pavlova. My cousin, the Norwegian princess, my friends from my new art class, and other local m8s – a whole array of good people came along. I didn't invite any of my exes, to make sure I felt free and independent. There was no pressure with any dressing code. Everyone came as they were and were happy for me. I loved the mixture of ages, races, classes and all. Within the usual lots of loving cards and presents, there was the most beautiful, silk, colourful scarf, which reveals my character very well: versatile, dynamic, warm, soft and shiny.

It was a good party because I was available for my friends, very happy to get to know their close ones. I really enjoyed being single myself, not tied to one person, therefore available and free to mingle and jingle in various ways. I enjoyed some deep conversations and also got a great BJ and made good use of my silver tongue in the toilets with a beautiful long-clitted stripper. She wanted more but I wanted to go back to my friends. My hero brother Matt was there entertaining everyone with his fantastic dancing skills and smiles, wearing and then losing my hat. Everyone enjoyed his company and discovered the real Matt, as I have always known him to be a flamboyant fun-loving, great dancer, a complete and utter star of the show, never showing off but just being and living each moment to the full. Watching him having so much fun and seeing everyone loving him and enjoying his company was a tonic to my evening.

I can say that this evening was the greatest birthday I have ever had. My mum agrees, as it is the first time I got home in a safe and rather healthy mood. This night proves my theory that a birthday resembles the year that has just passed and marks the vibe of the year that cometh.

Indeed, everything fell into place this year with me falling into a wheelchair: having to be pushed around changed my whole identity, becoming more looked after, which I never liked, losing all independence. On the other hand, the wheelchair also brought me more compassion, understanding and respect. Before the wheelchair, people who didn't know me would easily think that I was drunk because of my natural high and very strange way of walking. Now they just feel very much attracted by someone happy and loving who has risen above the prison of a wheelchair.

However, a few days after this wonderful party, I felt even more trapped than before in the comfort of my own home with my parents judging every one of my steps. I flew away again and got pissed and high. Of course, it caused my parents worry and anguish, even though my mum understands my need for independence. When I escape, I know I am free from boundaries and I don't care. Afterwards, I felt like a silly-billy teenager and a bit annoyed with myself. But the feeling of independence is stronger and more liberating than the pride of being mature. Being stuck at home can be a torture.

I believe that if I was independent in my own existence, I would be more responsible and build my own boundaries rather than having them pushed upon me.

However, I cannot live my own existence without some support. I need someone to help at home with cleaning, and eventually shopping if I didn't have a shop close to the flat. The best would be to live next to a shop, cinema and art gallery … I would be able to get so tired that it wouldn't matter that I didn't have the energy to pull myself out. If I fall down, I can get myself up, even if it takes time. I have accepted that. However, I may need a special application on my mobile to press a button in case of emergency. It may be good to have someone visiting every day just to make sure I'm OK. Or to share a house with other people in need of some support.

I don't think I would feel lonely and robbed of a life.

Mostly I need the PAs' support to bring important physical and creative activities and proper structure into my life.

Chapter 5

Dealing with MS at 38

More symptoms

At the same time as losing my balance, I also lost the good use of my eyes to read and it's getting worse, like everything else. Fortunately, I can see everything very well, except small details, especially when they are in line or in order. I can easily identify letters separately but they all get jumbled up when they're set together in words. My eyes jig about when I try to focus on small things put in line. It is so exhausting to read that I've just stopped that activity completely. Sometimes, when I'm a little better, I can suddenly read a bit again; I just have to go with the flow of what is left of me.

However, I can easily follow the ball making its way around the TV screen. Actually, I'm in a different place when I'm watching a football match; I long to be in there, knowing I should have been there scoring the winning goal. I am extremely focussed on every single player's action, with an overall vision of the game. I can see how I would play my part, and that hurts very much. At the same time, I am back to that joy I felt when I'd watch the games with my dad at White Hart Lane, but now I also feel a big void, missing the reality of actually playing a game. I was so obsessed by football as a kid, I loved Gary Lineker who now presents Match of the Day on BBC 1.

That could have been a great follow-up to my career as well, especially as football has became bigger than ever. Football has become so crucial to people who have found in it the power of belonging to a group, now that trade unions have less impact. Not only has the power of money and the media unfairly corrupted the face of football, but it has also made it one of the most meaningful things people have in their lives. It has also taken away from people the most important meaning in life, which is, for me, feeling and giving love. Basically, football also corrupts the feeling of love. The true love for a team and co-supporters and the need to belong to a group are exploited as a marketing tool. It's even worse that love can quickly become a caricature of hate. I don't miss the hooligans but they can raise their ugly faces at any time. Even the most violent animals don't behave like that.

It's funny how the illness changed my obsession from goals to girls. It also produced a deeper man than I thought I would ever become. I am sure that if I had become a famous footballer, I would have had quite a lot of girls as well, as many as George Best. I would have certainly fallen into the jet-setting star life-style, probably copying Vinnie Jones and maybe becoming an actor or a TV presenter. But I would also have put a lot of money into charities and supported my mother's generosity. I'd have liked to have been able to put money into a creative, inclusive organisation so that my brother Matt could also become a movie star and go to Hollywood. And I would have helped with all family members' dreams.

Back to MS reality. Writing is becoming more and more difficult. I can feel the pen between my fingers but I don't have complete control of drawing lines and forming shapes: nothing is smooth and coordinated, as it used to be. It is very slow and looks insecure with sharp angles. Strangely, my handwriting used to be like calligraphy, very regular and beautifully soft. Now it has become as erratic as a scribble, which makes me very upset, especially when I'm starting to enjoy becoming an author. And again, it's also exhausting; so exhausting that I don't even write anymore.

I used to be Mister Safe Hands and never dropped anything. I was excellent at cricket, playing in the Second XI at school. Now I can't hold anything in my hand safely, as the feeling of the object is not permanent or consistent. For instance, when I bring a cup to my mouth, I can lose the feeling of it between my fingers and can't control it slipping to one side and its contents running down on my shirt. Same with food. I don't really care about looking dirty but my entourage does, so I now need to wear an apron to eat. I feel like I am a five-year-old kid again and I laugh about it, but it still hurts.

The first symptom, of not feeling ejaculations, has spread out to most of my body. Fortunately, I can still feel my erections sometimes when I wake up in the morning or when I use Viagra. I am told that not having long-lasting erections anymore is just natural.

Losing my balance and sensory feelings goes with my loss of memory. It started after one of those break-ups when I was in my early thirties. I realised that I was losing my short-term memory as well as my photographic memory. I used to remember my ex-fiances' numbers by heart. Now I forget acquaintances' names. When I learnt something well, such as physics, I used to be good at; it doesn't mean much to me anymore and I'm not even interested in it, like many things that have been put out of my brain. Is it because they're not useful to me and my neurons are busy protecting me from any more harm? I still remember things that have affected me, such as my various love stories. Writing the book has helped me to revisit points in my life that I thought I had forgotten. I realise that memories are very important to recall so as to be able to identify yourself. Writing this book is fruitful in reviving my photographic memory and old feelings for things that used to inspire me.

Pills, doctors and counsellors

I have been on pills for almost 20 years for mind stabilisation. That has always been a good reason in itself to ingest other kinds of drugs to feel at ease.

Professor Kopelman is the finest doctor I have ever had; he is my ally. He is a neuropsychiatrist and seems to have all the mind skills. I met him when I was 19, on a day I will always remember as when my bipolar syndrome was diagnosed. Before that day, doctors only noted down my troubles and gave me various pills that would only calm me down for five minutes. When I met Professor Kopelman, I felt very relaxed in his company and quite trusting. I already knew that he was one of the heads of the psychiatric unit. I still visit him once every three months for a check-up and to renew my medication. He is my professor, with an 18-year relationship; he is the medical person who understands me best and I totally rely on his wisdom. He is such a cool dude.

He was quite surprised by my sexual life and tried to encourage me to stay in one relationship. But he knew that I was out of control and he didn't try very hard to master me, but rather give me some pills to level me out and make sure my mum could relax a bit. He did mention a couple of times that my drug-taking was dangerous for my condition, but I didn't care. He is the one who saved my mental health in giving me Carbamazepine in the first place. I am still on it, with 700 mg a day, which is half of the dose they were giving me ten years ago, when I was really uncontrollable. So, these pills did quite a good job. Whenever I forgot to take them, I got high as the sky within a day and would be out late that night, getting even higher with all kinds of other, illegal drugs and getting shags.

There are still big notes all over the house about the pills, to make sure I don't forget them, and my parents want to actually see me taking them. I feel those pills changed my level of energy, they take me down and can kill my spontaneity but they didn't change my character. I take a handful of pills all at once, twice a day. I don't even need any liquid to help them go through to my stomach because I have always a lot of saliva in my mouth, hence silver-tongued cavalier. It seems that I don't get many of the side-effects that most people get from Carbamazepine. It's difficult to know how much my other symptoms are due to that medication or to MS, or to know how much it exacerbates my MS symptoms.

My fatigue and my balance are definitely not aided by the chemicals. I have also always felt that this medication was the reason for my inability to ejaculate inside a lady and for my everlasting erection. I believe those chemicals enjoyed playing around with my sexual, godly nature, as much as the other substances I was using. Strangely, I never discussed those issues with my doctors. The beautiful nurses and psychologists around them would distract me from them. However, when my erection got affected, I didn't hesitate to talk to Kopelman about it, to have prescriptions for Viagra. I was so used to taking various types of chemicals that it seemed absolutely normal for me to take Viagra, in high doses as well. Now I know that high levels of drug-taking are probably the main culprits for affecting my erection, together with MS and age.

Anyway, I feel protected by Professor Kopelman's scientific and human knowledge. I would trust him with my life. He also gets on very well with my mum. She would come and talk with him after our one-to-one session. She is the one who told him about my overdosing on Viagra when I had only mentioned the business I was doing with it.

My specialist MS doctor from the hospital is another good ally. He has been by my side right from the start of this whole journey as a neurologist, since I was diagnosed with encephalitis, treating all my various symptoms at that critical time. Since then he has seen me regularly at least twice a year, advising, referring me to other specialists and writing letters to various social and health support services to try to get me help for my various issues.

Thanks to him and Professor Kopelman, lots of different people have been appointed to come to aid my good self. For instance, he found the right people to take care of all my body's plumbing issues (I have to pee as often as someone with prostate problems and I don't mention the other evacuation difficulties, as my bowels are no longer in good form), my sight, general neurological challenges, etc. He is a nice fellow and I enjoy seeing him every three months or so.

Both doctors have heard almost everything about my love life and were very interested about it. Of course, they are completely aware of how much my mania is helping to cope with my neurological condition.

It is quite unusual and I feel lucky about it, although my family is not that lucky to have to deal with me and the other symptoms that are happening. Mum has looked into the genetic history of the family to understand why we have gathered so many different illnesses, but she didn't find anything.

Interestingly, at the moment, progressive MS does not have any new drugs. There are many new drugs on the market for early stages of MS. But all have side-effects which are worrying. This is why we don't know how much Carbamazepine can affect MS. So we tried to reduce Carbomazepine a few times to better care for my neurological disease; unfortunately my mental state would come back to haunt me and I would run away to escape the trap of my existence. I know that if I took a few less pills, my balance would get much better. I could be a good subject for a medical study. I'd love to be paid to be a research object as well as entertaining a beautiful student. My mum would always find an excuse for me not to do that, because she protects my reputation. She is now wondering about the consequences of this book.

However, I realise I have been very lucky to keep my doctors all these years, when I haven't been able to keep a girlfriend or a therapist.

I started to see a therapist as soon as bipolar started taking over my life. I don't remember much about those sessions, I just know I didn't like them because it was only about my pain. Why would I enjoy turning the knife in the wound and how could that help me? Or it was about digging into the past, which was also painful when talking about my football times, and it seemed useless, as it had nothing to do with the actual MS issues. It is a waste of time and money.

Doing the same kind of work for this book is like being in a completely different dimension, as I'm leaving a trace and talking to the world rather than just talking to a boring therapist. Those therapists were not very amusing, even if sometimes I could get along with them. It's much more exciting to try to find the right words and to make them sound true as well as dark and fun, all at once, to catch the attention of an audience. It gives more sense to my life than giving it all to a dull therapist who is paid a fortune to listen to me. Also, I didn't feel like talking about the joys of sex with them; it seemed that a hospital room wasn't fitting, and someone paid by the government wouldn't be open to that. It would probably be easier with a French therapist and their psychoanalytical obsessions about sex. Moreover, I love to make love so much that I don't feel like talking about it to a therapist, as if it was a disease and a part of my condition.

I did enjoy talking about myself for a short while and then got bored with it.

The only session I remember was the one where I fell asleep. I was probably stoned as much as bored. I was obviously not the right kind of client, because I would always turn their questions around, back to them, rather than digging into myself for a deep answer that I already knew anyway. Whatever the reason, they would stop the therapy after a few sessions, saying it wasn't going anywhere. If they had been private therapists receiving £100 an hour minimum, they would certainly have found me extremely interesting and never stopped the therapy. I never tried to fuck any of them, which shows that I am not that idiotic. They would have loved it, but I wouldn't go in that direction, just because I didn't want to have a relationship with a counsellor. *Full stop*!

However, I have managed to make love to a few psycho professionals, who weren't my own therapists. I enjoyed that very much, because I could talk about very personal things with them, including the weirdest fantasies. We would normally portray those and they would enjoy developing their own. One had this fantasy to make love on the tube and so we did, on the Bakerloo line, very late on a Monday night. It was not empty but not full either. She had brought her own KY jelly because she also wanted it up the ass, and so we did. She had the most powerful orgasm. Then she sucked me off and then I went down on her with my silver tongue. A few people came and watched; I didn't mind at all. It excited me even more when a young couple came and took private seats and encouraged us verbally. They started to kiss and touch as well, but didn't get as hard as me and the psychotherapist. No one complained; it was free, live porn. I enjoyed it so much that I did it several more times with other women. Every time, we rocked the tube. I definitely helped women to discover their own fantasies.

I remember going to the cinema with another psychotherapist, but the movie was such rubbish that she went down on me. We weren't planning it but fortunately we were the only ones sitting in the back seats. The cinema usher came in, saw the blowjob was taking place and left with a big smile on his face.

I understand that therapists can be very useful to a lot of people, but for me it doesn't really work. I'm not waiting for them to change my condition, just to help me accept it and eventually move on from oral obsessive disorders such as sucking and licking. Again, writing this book is the best therapy, so read on! Actually, those therapists loved to hear my story so much that they have certainly unconsciously encouraged me to work on this book and to explore and write about my fantasies.

Regression

My bowels and my bladder cannot function normally. I have lost control of the bladder muscles and sometimes need to pee as often as every 15 minutes. It isn't always easy to find a place to pee within one minute and I often end up wetting myself. My mum has to drain me with a self-catheter before I go out. I have my pride and cannot behave like a tiny baby and let my mum do all the work. It's more a team work, where I hold my penis while Mum puts a narrow tube into it all the way up to my bladder. In a way it's quite lucky that I don't feel my penis, or this draining process would hurt me a lot. My Mum used to be a nurse and had seen all that before, plus she is definitely the closest person to me in the universe, since the day I was conceived. But having her checking on my adult penis still feels like I lack privacy and reminds me that I'm a disabled individual.

I know that I'll need that kind of support all my life and have to have a stranger do that to me if I want to live outside the family home. Moreover, Mum is getting old and she won't be my personal aid forever. She may need a personal assistant for herself one day. I am ready for a less comfortable dependency. We have a special toilet chair on the ground floor so I don't need to climb the stairs when I'm desperate to go to the loo. I always go out with a special bottle in my allocated bag. When I'm sitting on the bus, I can quickly open my zip and do a pee in the bottle, putting a little towel over my penis to cover my modesty, hiding behind my PA or the person accompanying me standing next to me. However, if anyone is watching, I don't care. I even enjoy telling people what's happening. It gives me a little buzz to share my misery. It's also quite exciting to have a pee in a public zone and risk having ladies watching. My other piece of luck is that my pee doesn't smell. So even if I wet myself, my chair and my trousers, it doesn't stink at all. That's why I wear dark trousers.

In relapsing periods, I also wet my bed at night. The idea of having to wear nappies has encouraged me to stay alert and take time to grab the bottle before flooding my bed. It seems this happens especially after I've have had an escape into drugs. Mum says it takes me a month to fully recover from an evening out binging.... Now it happens more often than not, without any drug-taking, so I've had to give in to my mother's advice for me to wear protectors (we don't call them nappies, I'm not a child). I know it's better for me. I don't need to piss myself. Although I am feeling protected, my pride is affected. Of course, I wish I didn't have to wear these protectors. Not as much as I wish I could still play football....

Fortunately, bowel accidents are not that frequent, even though I'm not a tight ass. Sometimes I don't even feel my sphincter. Therefore, it may happen that I find a big piece of shit falling from my trousers. I am quite lucky that most of the time it is dry and doesn't smell either. I am blessed in that fashion. Maybe I could use my dung in my art like Nigerian artist Chris Ofili.

Sometimes I go for a piss and a shit suddenly appears. It's interesting to see how much I can transform these humiliating handicaps into funny snags. My manic chuckling personality helps me to cope with these symptoms. I cannot blame anyone, therefore I'd rather laugh about myself and my childlike condition with a big penis and a humongous beard. However, when wet faeces are splashing around, I feel very human, but so abashed that I behave as if nothing has happened. Especially as, I can't clean it up myself, I prefer to ignore it and, trying to escape it, I just manage to spread it around the corridors. I know that my private situations can invade others and that makes me feel fiercely embarrassed.

However, I can only rest upon my chest and last a day before I go to sleep to a pure place where nothing is bothering me. My very deep sleep is another blessing. I never remember my dreams. Sometimes I feel that my soul has been robbed from me even though I know it is only my body … I exercised so well when I was young. I had a six-pack and everything.

I still try to exercise a lot now. Doing all kind of sports, especially for my legs, doesn't always seem to change things much; it just keeps the muscles alive, which is still helping my balance. I go three times a week to the gym with a PA or my mum, doing all kinds of machine-supported exercises. I stay for an hour or an hour and a half. This is the maximum I can work out before I get too exhausted. I used to go to the cinema after the gym, but it's a waste, as I fall asleep in front of the screen. I also go cycling in various places, using those great side-by-side bikes. Battersea park is the best place, not only for its natural beauty but also for all the beautiful women in shorts … I also go cycling to the velodrome by the same bus I used to take to go to school. I also sometimes go to the disabled cycling sessions in the park, where I gather with all kinds of very wacky people, sometimes with worse frailties than mine. This is when I know that I have moved to an unrecognisable world from where I was 20 years ago. I accept it because my family or my PAs are always there with me, as a solid link to normality. Plus, my friendly ways help me mingle well, which stops my loneliness and enhances my new identity.

My oral obsession is also getting worse, as I need to suck something all the time. But I am not a sucker. It is rather my denied silver-tongue existence that needs to find an outlet. It annoys my mother a lot because I look like a child sucking a dummy.

Relapsing periods

These come suddenly and clamp down my left leg and foot all at once, as authorities do with cars. It is caused in the right-hand side of my brain and travels across onto the left-hand side of my body. Then I also get extremely tired. I have noticed a couple of signs announcing a relapsing period, such as going to the loo every five minutes even if I don't have any girl waiting for me there, as it used to be.

Relapsing periods can last two days, two weeks or two months. My left leg is getting worse than it has ever been. It doesn't want to move. Each step is a great effort. The right foot is working fine; the left one has gone to sleep. My left leg was the first target of my diagnosed encephalitis and it is still the main one at each relapsing periods. For instance, sometimes my balance has been so bad that I couldn't even move my left foot up to climb the stairs. I had an accident that may have stopped the relapse. Entering the kitchen, my stick slipped, probably because I'd put too much weight on it at once; I tripped from the entry of the kitchen to the oven, as there was no other support to be grabbed, and I fell head first onto the grill, breaking the glass that exploded all over the kitchen and denting the metal panel.

As usual, I didn't feel hurt; my heavy bones easily supported the shock and my skin didn't show any kind of scar. Me and my people sometimes wonder from which planet I am from! My body is so weak but so strong at the same time, and my brain as well. I guess it is part of the multiple effects of the illness. The next day after that event, I felt much better with my balance and I could walk the stairs again. Internally, I could feel that the relapsing cloud was lifting from me. I wondered if the shock to the head had helped. Actually, it may have shaken my frontal lobe, as I feel so much better and calmer now.

Unfortunately, this relaxing moment didn't last more than a day and I went straight back to the old Charlie with a numb left leg and foot – that same foot that could bang goals into the top corner. My mum sometimes has to help my foot to climb each step. We now have another kind of push-chair that I use to walk across the kitchen to my favorite smoking spot in the garden. It is a mobility walker with brakes and a little seat I can put things on as I cannot push the chair and carry things around. It's amazing how many products are on the market for people with disabilities, so much that the price of them has dropped. I wish we didn't have to do research on that kind of product, but that's life.

Strangely, I am not permitted to have hot baths, as it can provoke a relapsing attack. The heat on my head is bad for my condition. It messes with my state of mind. Therefore, I am the fourth and last person in the family to have a bath, just to make sure it can't be hot. For the same reasons, I also have to be careful not to stay in the sun, even though I love it. My skin loves it too and gets a nice tan very quickly.

The cold also triggers my illness but the problem is that I cannot feel it at all. My nerves don't tell my brain about cold. So I love to think I am a firedragon that can beat the cold better than anyone. Unfortunately, my body hates it without letting me know. My entourage has to warn me about it all the time: 'Wear a jumper or a coat'. And again, I feel like a child whose firedragon destiny is being denied.

Sharing with disabled people

Instead of accommodation away from home, the social services are at least offering me an opportunity to leave the house once a week and start enjoying the company of disabled people. It is good to have this first experience with them before I may be sent to live with them full time in a care-home or in sheltered accommodation. Every Thursday a coach comes to pick me up, together with a bunch of six to ten other people, to go and have a laugh in a nice centre. We first have coffee and cake and some of us share a cigarette outside. There is a computer room where I don't go because I have my own computer at home anyway. I go to their gym room for a bit of a work out. Sometimes we can play pool, but as you can guess I cannot play pool so well anymore.

So, basically, we are mainly there to chat and spend time together. Nobody talks about their own personal strife, except me. So a few people have come up to me to tell me they also have MS. Most people enjoy my bubbly personality; they come and connect with me with eyes and a smile, if not with words. We can also have some interesting conversations, whatever their education and culture. It took me a little while to appreciate their company. I was at first perturbed to be put in a box with disabled people After a few months I realised I enjoyed their company and the more I see them the more I get to know them and find them cool. Even those who dislike me.

I can tell from their eyes and behaviour and from what other people tell me that I am an annoying figure in their life. They touch my hand in an aggressive way. I know I behave as if I don't care but I don't know yet how to change my behaviour to please everyone. So I just put those negative feelings in the back of my mind. That's something I can do much better than hushing my noise. I'm afraid that is what mania is about ... I believe I am the youngest and probably considered to be the craziest, and for sure the most talkative. Even if I feel that I am a kind of animator to the group, I really appreciate the fact that we are all on the same level, carrying all kinds of heavy debilitating loads.

There is much respect and solidarity within the group. I wouldn't mind living with some of these individuals in a shared home if I could have my own private space. Basically, it's good to have a day out from my comfortable prison, with a bunch of friends who are easy to talk to, and away from stress. However, sharing some time with very disabled people is helping to accept the man I am becoming. They are a vision of my struggle and my inner self. I can have glimpses of what my future can become if I don't look after myself. I am very moved by the people who can't talk properly. For instance, a man with four children and grandchildren cannot talk very well, although he can think very clearly. I cannot stand the idea I could lose my voice or my ability to talk. I would feel castrated. That would be a nullification of my life, even though my smile would never leave my face and I may have more friends if I shut up or am just quieter.

Seeing people who are more disabled than me gives me a positive mental attitude; I can see my own fortune and capability better than usual, and they give me the will to work harder on myself. Enjoying their company also helps me to accept myself in that disability box.

I also like the way the employees are with us. They are completely on our side. The gym worker pushes me and my legs right to the top biking level. We have an agreement that I will go and stay with him in his home country in South America when we win the lottery. I also got 'engaged' to a beautiful gym lady who is also doing the bible class. Those professional carers accept my funny ways better than most and know how to put limits on my behaviour in a nice and professional manner. If they saw me every day they may be less caring.

We all connect on a level unknown to many – the strain of total dependency, together with the joy of feeling unique and of being able to share and give, even if it's just a smile. Nevertheless, I haven't found a significant other there.

My deepest pains

Indeed, giving and making love is what I miss most, aside from playing football as well as I did. Since my last love left to study away from London, it has been years without any intimacy with a woman. I know it isn't the end of it and I will make love a lot in the future. I can still wank and come, but I never feel much. The best thing about wanking is the fantasy, thinking about the ladies I made love to (BIB is still the best one).

However, even if I cannot feel my prick inside a woman and I cannot feel an orgasm, I can feel her coming. I can definitely see it coming first in her eyebrows; this is why I love eyebrows so much, because they can express more than words and even more than thoughts. I can tell from the faces and noises she makes. I really miss those times – yes, the woman's orgasm is what I miss most.

One of the most hurtful feelings is not to have any children, especially as quite a few women desperately fantasised about having a baby with me. I may have quite a few children around but none of those possible mums would seriously want me as a father. I understand there are many reasons for that and I accept it. It was not meant to be for me. It is probably much better like this, as the poor child would have had two parents on benefits and a dad often acting like a child. Not sure all this would have given the child the opportunity to shine, especially as our so-called non-judgemental liberal society would decide on his or her education and placement in a foster family rather than staying with his loving parents.

However, I'm lucky that I'm able to procreate until I die. I'm sorry for the ladies; men tend to win on that factor. So, I can just hope I will become a father one day. Hope is my drug, but I have to be realistic on the matter. There would be several positive sides to my possible parentship. First, I would not be running away from home to go to work and would be available for the child to give him or her love and attention all day. I would be playing with him/her a lot, teaching him/her love and respect, encouraging his/her creativity, teaching art, laughing and dreaming a lot.

I suffer from my dependency on the government, who can decide what is good for me. Because I'm entitled to benefits, they have a tendency to think they know what my needs are and they are authorised to take control of my life. This is a true vicious circle where health/social services can oppress people. I am very lucky I have a mother who fights for my rights and is always researching for me to find my way in dignity (and for herself to get a bit more freedom). She also believes she knows what my needs are, but I trust her so much. She made sure that we were able to access the Social Service's Direct Payments that allow us to make some decisions by ourselves. Thanks to her, I sometimes feel that I am in control of my own life. I love her. She is always there for me and always tells me that if I respect myself and others I will be respected back. If I were in the US, I would probably be a homeless drug addict on the street or in prison. I am well aware of how much our British government deals with the fate of vulnerable people.

The worst pain is not being able to control my life and my body. I used to have the perfect career in front of me, with the finest body, and then the perfect erection. Now all I think about is what I used to have. The only thing I have left is to dream of a happy future and I hang on to that dream as if it is real. I believe I am going to be rich and famous! This book will sell so many copies worldwide and a film will be made. No one is sure about this except me. At least I can control my dreams. I even hang on to the fact that my MS could disappear. People don't believe me and they don't understand that belief is a crucial ingredient of my existence.

Another way to compensate for the lack of control is to control the few people around me by ordering them around and believing they should be 100 per cent available for me. I only realise this is an idiotic way of behaving when my parents tell me off ferociously. That is how I know I am very wrong because my parents are such gentle souls. Unfortunately, that behaviour is another thing I can't control. I don't *think* before I ask. Especially with Mum, as we are so close. And with my PAs, we're pushing each other around; they push my wheelchair and I push their patience. It's different with Mab, who writes this book with me: she pushes my brain and I enjoy that very much.

Art and my struggle

Strangely, I have rarely felt inspired to express my frustration and pain through art, even though it always does come through. It was only right at the beginning of my struggle that I made work directly associated with my illness. It is definitely beauty and joy that I want to communicate about, but sometimes it is overtaken by the pain. MS has never helped me build myself as an artist, even though I had so much time available. I used to be good at drawing things until I couldn't always feel the pencil on the paper. It's the same when I'm walking and I can't really feel my feet. In fact, I can't feel the resistance of the ground nor the paper. It's the same when I drop things.

But those feelings, or rather lack of feeling, can come and go; it isn't steady. Therefore, I can never trust myself. I can never tell if I am going to have a good or a bad day, with good or bad balance and use of my hands. It is quite basic and physiological but it is also losing control of myself, which is mentally very very tricky and difficult. I have no other choice than to go with the flow and accept being in my own chains. Actually, I used to feel that my soul was creating itself through my hands. That no longer exists, except the feeling of being creative. The internal powers and wisdom are inspired by the beauty surrounding me.

We tried different other avenues, so that I could keep on expressing myself through the arts and nurture my love for creation and beauty. I tried printmaking and have been able to produce some brilliant work. But since I depend on other people to do most of the technical work, my lack of concentration doesn't allow me to be as agile with my creativity. It is difficult for me to dig into the piece of art and get visual thoughts moving in the way they used to. It is probably this frustration that made me react with loudness and disturb the last printmaking art class I went to. I was showing off because I had got nothing much to show. But nobody dared tell me to shut up, certainly because I'm in a wheelchair.

They excluded me from the course in a bizarre fashion. It came as no surprise to me, as I've been excluded from so many courses in London, which I am not proud of. But this time, they didn't even blame my usual disturbing behaviour; they didn't even dare talk to me directly about it. They just wrote to my mum saying I was not able to take advantage of the teaching. It shouldn't have been the main point, as they knew that I wasn't technically and creatively alert and mindful. They have not dared to tell me the truth – to shut my mouth – because of my disability. I guess I get what I deserve: they didn't treat me as a sensible person, because I'm not sensible when I'm in class. It is probably both the potential creative freedom – which I can't reach anymore – and the influence of the group on me. There were quite a few nice ladies who I took a shine to. However, I would really prefer it if people dared to tell me to pipe down. Please do be honest with me; I need to be reminded regularly about all boundaries.

Now I am going to art college again – one of the rare colleges that never excluded me. But not being able to do printmaking and photoetching anymore, I am booked in to the drawing and painting course. We draw with charcoal, which is much easier for me than with a pencil. Painting is the easiest and the most liberating form of art. I can just play with the colours, mixing them up, creating some new ones, jollying around with texture and movement, and the outcomes can be stunning. I feel much freer than at the printmaking class and I am focussing more, especially as my mum is often there with me, helping and shutting my mouth up so I don't disturb the class.

I can't flirt, either. Quite boring, as art and women have always been linked for me. It's strange not to be inspired by sex and lust as I used to be. However, I still enjoy the creative process a lot, expressing the visual whims going through my mind. It looks like the presence of my mother is waking up some Oedipus complex to sort out my art inspiration!!!!!! She loves what I am doing and I enjoy following her suggestions. The fusion is still there between us and fills me with creative energy. Because my mum needs a rest, it is now wonderful to have an old school friend as a personal assistant. As I said before, she is my favourite assistant, as she helps bring the best out of my creativity. Painting makes me feel a real zest for life – indeed, as much as going out and about with like-minded people.

I have always had time for art throughout my life, as well as for the ladies, and for me now, painting brings back those memories, especially in art college where I spent some of my most creative and sexy times. It is like a second home to me and I love to go there. The other students at the college – those that don't have a disability anyway – must have a very different experience of the place than I do. They arrive, go to their class, interact with their tutor and other students and then go home. As I access the building in a different way, it has enabled me to meet the people who run it, behind the scenes, and that has been a real positive.

Sometimes the lift is out of order and I have to be assisted up a flight of stairs by a couple of members of staff. This makes me sad, as I never used to need anyone's help, but asking for help is a very real thing in my life now. It has to be done; it's just the way it has to be now. The real positives of this are the college facilities staff who help me. The people who work there are very special and I'm sure most other students don't get to meet and chat to them like I do. Especially the building manager is a brilliant man. He is always on the ball, has a great sense of humour and he's now a good friend to me. The other staff are incredibly cool and it's a pleasure to know them all.

Most importantly, the tutor is the most amazing I have ever had. I think we both relate to one another, both being talented artists. We get on very well, understanding each other's humour. He knows how to push me outside my comfort zone and gives me the kind of advice I need. My art has really improved since being taught by him. I really feel what I want to draw and paint and my tutor gives me the freedom to do that. He also knows how to hush my noise, with respect. I've always had a real feel for art but when I'm with people I trust I can really let things go and express myself. I love to produce work that people enjoy, and the class is great; it's full of lovely, supportive people who I love being with. I'm very happy to have a place to do my work. My tutor chose a piece of mine for the art exhibition. I felt so proud to see my art on the wall and people looking at it as they walked around. I'd love to have a big exhibition one day. The self-portrait I made in printmaking when I had just been diagnosed with encephalitis would be central to that, because it expresses all the confusion we were going through, carrying all my pain and the weight of my future.

I wish my illness allowed me to paint all the time. Before, art never tired me out; even if I was really tired, I always had energy to complete my work and feel good. It was the freest way I could express myself, rather than being a loud bar steward all the time! I wish painting still allowed me to get what's in my head out on paper so that afterwards I could feel relieved and light, as if I had finally been able to express the perplexity of my life. Here is a quote by Kitaj, when he had returned to drawing on his own brush with death and illness as a theme: 'Hemingway told Fitzgerald: "We are all bitched from the start, and you especially have to hurt like hell before you can write seriously. But when you get the damned hurt, use it".' As I can no longer use my hands so well to create, I am now using words to examine my life. It doesn't feel very arty, but it is a new way of creating. It is not such a natural way for me to express myself, so I need my ghostwriter, and enjoy having these words dug out of my brain. It feels like a great relief when they come out!

Hospital loves and dislikes

When I fall down hard or get a urinary infection or any other complication, I get hospitalised for a few days, or a few weeks or a few months until they put me back on track. This last time, I fell all the way down one full floor from my bedroom. As usual I didn't feel any hurt but I was moaning a bit because I knew I had hurt myself and was afraid the injury would take me to hospital. It happened that I had a urinary infection at the same time. So, I really had to go to hospital. The NHS is a dream place where they will take care of you for free when you are feeling so unwell. Actually, they had to keep me in hospital for two months just because they could not find a place in a physio rehab ward for me to recover my strength after a couple of weeks in bed. So here I am, stuck in a medical ward with very sick people, most of them in intensive care, all looking like freaks. My bed neighbour just seemed to be dying, constantly whining and calling out for help when he wasn't unconscious. His family was panicking around him. I felt so uncomfortable that I compensated by showing off my good health, talking a lot to the healthy people around.

As a matter of fact, it is amazing how things change for me as soon as I'm in a hospital bed, just because I am surrounded by nurses. So many women turning around me! There are about 20 of them supposedly taking care of me. I miss the family and my own space a lot but being taken care of is very much appreciated. I take all the opportunities to chat with these ladies who are there for me and I never hesitate to offer to get engaged to them, even on the first encounter. I flirt outrageously.

First, they say nothing and just smile; I enjoy taking that smile for a flirt back, which encourages me to pursue the flirting. Then they may eventually ask me to shut up, in a nice way, but it seems that they rather want to play the game a bit further. They enjoy the chat and the compliments but refuse to hear about the hot stuff. I keep on telling everyone that I love them, including my neighbours on the ward, and they tell me they love me as well, which is nice even if they don't mean it.

I can see that the nurses enjoy me asking personal questions, even if they often don't dare answer. Some of them really enjoy chatting through my fantasies for a minute, then back out and we go on at their next visit with the next chapter of that fantasy. I enjoy it when they play these games with me. It has always been my dream to have a nurse in my boudoir and it would help to make me feel at home and to be taken care of. (There is an interesting link with the fact that my mum is qualified as a nurse …).

However, I quickly miss feeling a bit active. After a few weeks, my infection has been well treated and the tests show no injury after my fall down the stairs. I just feel like myself again and want to go home and to be able to move around and do my own thing, go back to art and the gym routine with my lovely PAs. Here in this hospital I feel like I'm in prison for no reason. Nobody has told me why I'm stuck here. It's hard enough to be disabled; it's much harder to be treated like a disabled old sick guy when I feel on good form. Anyone who's in prison for no reason would feel angry and hurt by this entrapment.

It's so unfair that I start feeling paranoid. I have the feeling my mum is happy to have me here. As a matter of fact, it is certainly easier for my parents without me at home – especially when they are just in the middle of major works, as the ground floor of the house is being refurbished to install my new suite.

The NHS and social services have finally realised that my mum can't physically support me going upstairs. We're very lucky to have been given a grant from our council to be able to keep me in my own home and within my own community. So, while I am in the rehab centre my parents have managed to turn the whole house upside down so they can get that suite built in what was the sitting room. A great architect designed it with a lovely accessible bathroom and my own private access to the garden.

The strange thing is that I cannot even tell Mum how I'm feeling about being stuck here in hospital. How come I cannot express such basic needs to my own mother? I have no problem telling all that to Mab, who comes to visit me once a week, and letting her talk to Mum about it. I feel very hurt to believe that the family is happy about my absence. This may be the reason why I can't talk about all this. Being away from Mum while being in good health hurts me more than if I was sick and needing care. I may have appreciated being taken care of and regressing a bit more than usual, but after a while and being so healthy again makes me feel like running away. My escape fantasies are coming back big time.

Fortunately, after Mab talks to my mother about my feelings, Mum manages to get a doctor to talk to me about my condition. As a matter of fact, I need quite a lot of physio before being able to go back home. I have lost muscle strength and I have to accept that I have also lost quite a lot of balance and control of my body. It pisses me off to realise I can't even stand up!! I have been in bed far too long! My family had been talking to me for months about the fact that I couldn't live in the room upstairs anymore, but I was so resistant about it. Now I have to face the reality: I'm in bed in hospital because I cannot live as I used to. I react as usual with my happy, funny, manic attitude, talking to everyone and maybe sounding foolish. Some nurses are not so patient with me anymore and believe I have the mind of a three-year-old, which is even more frustrating.

After a couple of months, the NHS finally manages to get me a bed at a really nice physio rehab place. It's like a four-star hotel, with big lovely airy rooms opening out onto a lovely garden. There is someone sitting next to me all day to make sure I don't stand up and fall down. It is quite amazing how they can spend citizens' money to protect vulnerable people to fit in their boxes, all at the right time.

One of the best outcomes of this whole experience has been that I have stopped smoking. Amazingly, it's like giving up a drug habit without the bad effects. The strangest thing is that I wasn't even thinking about it in the early days of not smoking and I'm not thinking about it anymore now, even when I go home for a day. Plus, I'm saving so much money! I think that stopping smoking helps me feel much better about myself, physically and mentally, and I believe that I can give up every bad habit now.

It seems that I'm dropping a few other oral habits, such as sucking everything. As I talk about it, I'm about to put something in my mouth, not because I need it but because I'm mentioning it. However, I am still an oral addict in that I am asking everyone here to give me a hot chocolate, because it is free at the common dining room and kitchen. Before they realised I was a sugar addict, I became quite fat. Looking back on my silly chain-smoking habits, I can't believe I was such a stupid idiot to try to kill myself that way.

I have physiotherapy every day for about 45 minutes. They make me stand up and walk under control. Otherwise, they make sure I don't walk at all to avoid me falling again, so I am stuck in my chair all day, or lying in bed. I'm peed off being stuck in my wheelchair!! I was definitely doing a lot more physio at home, walking around with my stick. They are really sweet people here but they're not letting me take any initiative, which I feel is very annoying. Also, like in hospital, they don't listen to me anymore. They know what I'm going to say anyway, as I have a tendency to repeat myself and I am told I am quite loud as well. It's difficult for me not to be the centre of attention and, as a compensation for being stuck in a chair, I like having people serving me.

I cannot wait to go back home and experience my brand-new suite and my hood.

It took two months for social services and the rehab centre to finally agree that I could go home. A social worker came and saw me several times at the rehab centre. He took great care to find out what I wanted and needed. After several assessments and many reports and panels, they realised how much extra assistance was needed for me to be able to go home. In the meantime, they kept on saying I would only have to stay for another couple of weeks. Was it a lie or was it to keep me going strong? They didn't have a clue, just like me. What a nightmare! Did they think that my memory loss was so bad that I would forget their announcement? It's like promising a kid a sweet or a treat to calm him down and then never giving it to him. That can make a kid furious and bitter.

It was the ultimate betrayal for me, treating me like a kid and expecting me to react like an adult. I was indeed feeling worse than a kid there: no one listening to me, having to repeat myself all the time and to shout so everyone gets really annoyed. The worse was having someone watching me 24/7. Someone was actually paid to sit next to me just in case I decided to get up and fall down. At first, I did enjoy having a presence, especially when I was in a single room. It helped kill my boredom. After a couple of weeks, it became a nightmare, as I realised nobody trusted me and I felt like a lion in a cage, watched by a guard. I have never attacked anyone but occasionally I would threaten to complain to their boss so that they would change their behaviour and do something to make up with me.

It took those long weeks for the social and medical services to agree on a good package of care for my decreased level of physical ability and for me to access the new home-suite fully. In the end it turned out that everything fell into place quite nicely. Thank you to the staff and to the social worker involved.

Released from prison at last

Now I am aware that if I had been able to realise my dream and leave the family home to live in a care home, it would be the same as here in this 'perfect rehab home': not able to take any initiative nor any risk, stuck with other people I have nothing in common with, constrained to patience, being a very passive young man and not being the cool cat. Mum and Mab also believe that in a care home, I would become so impatient and frustrated that I might erupt and become so loud and difficult that they might neutralise me with drugs. At home there are other controlling ways but they are from the people I love most. Mum is able to challenge me in her own way, and I can challenge her as well, which makes life a bit more exciting than being a very patient and passive frustrated patient. Most importantly, Mum has got my full trust now as I see how she challenged everyone to support my growth.

I am looking forward to my new home, my family and my new carers: it will be a new life, accepting that I cannot walk around anymore. No girlfriend in sight but quite a few lovely ladies to take care of me. I cannot have everything, can I?

The most satisfying emotion in getting home is probably to find my brother. I realise how I've missed him. We've rarely lived apart for so long. I had forgotten how intelligent and mature he is. First thing I do is to take him out for a coffee and ask him to tell me what has happened during my absence. I am so happy to hear that he missed me a lot as well. Here we are, the cool, eccentric pair of brothers. When people recognise me on the street, it feels so good to be myself again. Even a lady from a previous relationship recognised me; she was taken aback to see me in a wheelchair, she didn't have a clue of what to say or do. I flattered her and asked her about her new partner. She couldn't answer back but looked at me and smiled. We both remembered our last hot meeting and she said she would like to come and visit me again. I could tell it wasn't for sex anyway, even if I'd have died for sex with her again. Am I becoming as wise as my granddad??

I had seen my new suite a few times at weekends before leaving the rehab centre. I'd been able to choose the colours: pale yellow on the walls and blue bed cover and sofa, and some furniture. Now I am finally home, and that is what is most important; but I'm feeling reduced down from my top-floor boudoir to a ground-floor suite with direct access to the garden. I still wish it was a boudoir where lovely girls could have fun. I have to accept that it is not a very private romantic place. It is rather a homely sitting room with a medical bed which had to be extended to suit my tall size. This bed can be lifted up and down. During the first months back home, the bed had a kind of hoist and a piece of equipment called a 'cricket' to lift me from my wheelchair into bed. Mum had to have proper training to use it.

It could have been fun to be lifted in the air without any muscle effort and softly slam-dunked into bed, like a ball being chucked and easily scored into the back of the net, but I felt very heavy and disabled, never as easy to move around as a ball. It felt more as if I was still in hospital, needing so much help to do such a basic thing as go to bed. I didn't like this machine and tried a few times to get up on my own but heavily fell down on the ground, hurting my wrist and ankles. Also, the carers had to use it to lift me up on to the bed and change my pads. *I am not a baby.* These nappies piss me off! I know they are only pads and I have to accept that I cannot go to the toilet on my own anymore. However, it's quite relaxing and enjoyable not to have to rush to the toilets every 15 minutes and above all to let go all my waste, not having to control anything.

Now, after a few months back home, I've been able to build some strength back, going to the gym every two days for 45 minutes, and having physio exercises at home with carers and Mum. The physios' goals for me were to be able to stand up from the wheelchair so as be able to go to bed on my own; most of them had lost the belief that I could walk at least a few steps again. Nevertheless, Mum and I keep noticing the progress made, and to be made. Mum has to behave like a Rottweiler to push and convince the physio team to make me work harder. Now I still need a smaller cricket hoist and some help to go from the wheelchair to the cricket and then to transfer my big body from the cricket to the bed.

Carers from social services are now coming four times a day to check me out in everyway. They always come in pairs to be able to hold me up.

Two are coming in the morning at about eight to get me out of bed, into the cricket hoist, then into a shower commode and to the shower. I'm sitting in the shower commode while a male carer is scrubbing me down. I'm trying to dry myself off on my own. Then the carers put my pull-up nappies on, then I'm back to the wheelchair, and then they put my clothes on. They're coming back at about noon to see if I need a change of nappies and sometimes they serve me lunch. And then back at five and again at seven thirty to prepare me for the night. They are the same four carers coming every day. They seem to enjoy coming here, not only because they are always smiling and joking around; they also seem to enjoy taking a little rest on my sofa. They know how to push me around sometimes, encouraging me to move my big body, as I may be quite lazy sometimes, or asking me to stop calling for mum for everything. I can see it is difficult for some of them to understand my needs, especially my oral obsession, or get where I am coming from and how my brain is working. Being stuck in a wheelchair with an illness that makes me feel exhausted all the time doesn't help. Obviously when I'm on the street I'm all lively and out there again, full of beans and still ready to conquer the world.

I also have four PAs to come and take me out, to the gym, cinema, out and about on the Common, shopping, dining, etc. One lovely PA lady has been preparing us for a charity marathon, her running and pushing me in the wheelchair around the Common. The National Literacy Trust is this amazing charity that wants to give every kid the opportunity to learn to read, write and speak, no matter what start in life they may have had!! It has been really exciting to participate in helping improve the life chances of many children from deprived backgrounds.

We sent emails around to raise money for that race and there we went, two whizzy, wheeling and running people for the National Literacy Trust and all these disadvantaged kids!

Even though education didn't help me get the job/money/power that any young man would want because of my condition, I am aware that it gave me loads of clues as to who I am and the world I am in, and it participated in my self-esteem. It probably gave me a clearer understanding of priorities, and helped me put have some distance from the worries and burdens of life. Therefore, it was really good to be able to give back. We managed to raise £770, which happened to make us the best fundraisers of the event!!! I felt very proud to be doing this.

It was a cold and windy Sunday in March. Mum and the carers got me ready quite early. My PA and her mum picked me up to get there for ten o'clock. We were wearing the charity red-and-white striped tee-shirts with number 159 for me and number 121 for her. We were over 450 people running the 5k race (there was a child 1-k race and another adult 10-k race) and we arrived in 250th position, which I believe is great for pushing an average wheelchair with a 14-stone body sitting in it. We did it in about 40 minutes, which makes it 8 km per hour. F is a great runner with a natural fit body and she trains almost every day. I was trying to encourage her and was hearing her breathing hard. I was feeling a bit like a horse running in front of a carriage, although I was the carriage. It was so cool to be among all these people in doing something positive. I would love to do more things like that, so anyone who has a charity project that can include a wheelchair, I'm in!

It is hard to have to resign to others doing everything and at the same time it is great to have so many nice people taking care of me. I have to obey, and accept being dependent on the carer's schedule and the technical aids to support my big body. I've got used to complying and have learnt to see the advantages of it. At the same time, I make sure my needs are heard. One of them is to have so many lovely ladies taking care of me. Another is to have someone available almost all the time and to prevent my mum having to be there all the time.

An area where I have improved since being back home is the way I talk to ladies. It is much easier to get their attention when you compliment them and look them right in the eyes. I always knew how to do that and – lucky me – I still have my smiling eyes and cheeky attitude. I am now more careful and make sure I don't shock them with harsh talk or inappropriate gestures. I also punch and squeeze people less, and don't ask every woman in sight to marry me. However, I still long for a girlfriend and dream of finding one. Maybe this book will help me to seduce a wonderful lady.

Now Dad needs to be looked after more than me, as he broke his leg. It hurts, as he used to be the power behind most things in my life. We share the same carers, who keep busy like bees going from my front bedroom to the kitchen where a medical bed has been installed for Dad. The kitchen has been transformed into a lovely bedroom, facing the garden.

Chapter 6

Matters of acceptance

Love is the basis of it all. I know I have been blessed by love all my life. I thank the higher powers, whatever they are, for that gift. *Cheers*. Love is at the core of all religions and is the Higher Spirit I believe in; it can cleanse it all and grant a better future. Goodness is the key. However, I don't believe in an Almighty God, because I don't believe there is One Truth but I do respect everyone's own beliefs. There is a way for each individual to discover their own spiritual path according to their background and circumstances. They will find it eventually if they are looking for it.

Accepting who you are and believing in yourself are the most crucial ingredients for a happy life. If you can capture your own essence and know what is most important for you – some people call it values, and in my case, it is all about *love* – then you can thrive in your life on a good journey. Confidence is so crucial. I understand that my mental state is making me over confident, which is very helpful for me but can annoy other people. I am very much aware of this and I apologise for anyone I have bothered. However, confidence is completely different from arrogance. Do you know why? Confidence is from within; arrogance is from without.

Faith is so important for lots of people, it guides them and supports them in the bad times. But when it goes for only one truth and extremes, faith can become negative and even hateful, leading to war. Look at all terrorists! Or just at the people who only believe in money, status and good looks. They dismiss people who don't have what they possess or don't have the right look. I learnt from being unfaithful to my fiancée that when you truly love someone you should never stray. When you strongly believe in something or someone, you should just dig into your feelings or beliefs. If the feeling is real you will be able to feel its soul in a touch, a kiss or just a word. Nevertheless, the illusion of Love can become damaging in many ways. I remember breaking many girls' hearts and being myself dependent on various feelings that I thought were love. I do realise now they were not love but a physical lust or just a need for power and recognition. Becoming the master and not the slave definitely helped me not to give in to MS, although I am now completely aware that I *am* a slave to MS.

Some people can become slaves of love and get destroyed by their feelings. I'm a very lucky man because love has always been part of my life as a natural gift from my family. I didn't choose this soul-giving family, and my mum certainly didn't choose this path. Rather it seems that my life has been a journey to understand the various powers and illusions of love.

This is where my fantastic mother's contribution may come in to show again her unconditional love, patience, understanding and strength: my mum's amazingness taught me to believe in myself and be confident whatever happens.

> Charlie – my open tribute to you
> Charlie – you came into the world – the umbilical cord around your neck – bursting with energy – vigour – determination – and power. So beautiful – blond-haired – strong – tender – full of fun – naughty – bright – with friendship in the air.
>
> Layla and you – loved deeply by us – learning and exploring – both so accepting of Matt – valuing difference from the start.
>
> Charlie – so studious – thrilled by exploration – helpful – tender – shy – artistic and so skilled on the football pitch – your individual skill and art. So much potential.
>
> Fishing – swimming in the Usk – BBQ's under the stars – deep into the night – camping – riding – walking the Brecons – friendships – drinking – binge-drinking – football – football – football – Dad's pride of you – Spurs – dreaming – dreaming of being a star – teenage exploration – Invincible.
>
> Only 17 – a tingling – a life-change – steroids – blindness – so brave – so resilient – MS – relapsing – remitting MS – I will survive. Only 19 – MS/bipolar disorder – (remember amazing people have bipolar) – mental health the Cinderella of the health system.
>
> Deep challenges to your indomitable spirit. Carpe diem – Deep challenges – why me – depression – mania – MS – Bipolar – Fuck the world – fuck my parents – I will survive – how I want to survive – Silver-tongued cavalier – Deep challenges to us as a family – but with help we tried to understand – immensely supportive GPs – helped by other consultants – but especially Michael Kopelman – who gave you,

and us as a family, immerse respect and involvement in your treatment – and, most importantly, listened. From friends who stood by us all at times of immense stress.

Knowledge of the social model of disability and rejection of the medical model our stabilising force. Disabled friends so clear – invaluable insight – in-depth experience – inclusion the key.

Art colleges – girlfriends – deeper relationships – some easy – some disastrous – you were still trying to explore the scene.

Freedom – independence – let me be free. We tried to let you be free – no real knowledge what that meant other than independence – Danger – late-night collections from dubious places – strangers in the night – the comfort of being with others with similar addictions and thus being understood – Rejection – Fear and anxiety – Family – extended family confused – fear for our other wonderful children – denial of reality – bolstered by friendships – love and connection. We will survive – and we have.

Deterioration – MS progression – a fall – hospitalisation – fantasies – always dreaming – always believing that things will change – always positive.

For the moment you are at home – your own space – amazing agency carers who make this possible – direct payments – achieved by Disabled People's Campaign to be in control of their own lives – facilitating personal assistants who have become friends and extended and added so much to your life – and our life.

Your story with the help of Mab is remarkable, and a real tribute to your open honesty and loving nature. Mab has been your confident and stabiliser for five years – for which we thank her so much. I only hope that readers will understand the significance of the journey you have taken and the barriers you have had to overcome, including the effect that MS and its complications have on cognition and behaviour.

You are deeply loved, Charlie – by family and friends and advisors – admiring of your spirit – and ready to walk the walk with you always. Thank you for introducing us to such a diverse crowd of people, initiated by your capacity to include, love and believe in everybody – Thank you for opening our eyes to a journey we never expected – challenging us to our very being – but one which has made us love and admire you more than we can ever say – *Carpe Diem* – your Motherhood!!

I should be so angry at the way life is going, I was supposed to be a professional footballer and my life is melting away from me. I have been put into a box and a chair, because my whole body, brain and soul are distraught. There are many many many reasons for me to be angry, torn apart between so many realities and disabilities. I feel very restrained, diminished and tied down but I still never feel nor express any anger. Except some frustration sometimes towards my mum when she is over controlling and towards myself when I am too useless or if I hurt someone. Just like I don't feel physical pain, cold or burn, I do not feel anger. What's the point? It's a magical and spiritual, or just neurological, gift that was given to my mind, maybe by the doctors with those huge doses of steroids on my young brain; or is it just the illness that had that big effect on my frontal lobe and gave me the manic part of bipolarity??? I don't know. Je ne sais pas. I can just observe that the mental pain is drifting out of myself. Leaving free rein to my over-sexuality, and escaping into drugs has certainly not helped my double-whammy condition but was certainly a way to avoid the pain, whether it was anger or anxiety. Letting go does not mean giving up.

However, I loved that life to the full and I don't regret the consequences that I'm paying for now. Yet, not feeling the anger does not mean I'm denying the pain. I have been even more fully aware of it since writing this book, and my ghost writer is pushing me to face reality all the time rather than escape into my fantasies.

My strong and crazy soul does not allow the anger but it does let me express my torments, with a big smile on my face. People say it's bad to keep things trapped inside because they will hurt or kill you eventually. Or running away from them, they will catch you sooner or later. Talking to everyone on the street is my way to say, 'Check me, I'm alive and happy in my wheelchair, the man with a second face'. At home there has never been any barrier to talking about my issues. Therefore, the reason why I don't feel the anger may be also because I can express the pain. I can feel this is the only way to learn to accept it and to renounce normal existence, to let go of a champion and a life as a father.

When we started talking about all this for this book, I used to feel the urge to go and smoke, dope if possible. But as I cannot escape anymore, I am learning to confront it and accept it, as I put words to it and share it with the world. I also realise that it isn't that hard to live without power, sex and drugs and it isn't that painful anymore. Letting go is the hardest thing, but when you can achieve that and accept to renounce, you feel much stronger than ever as you discover a new power to control your urges rather than being controlled by them. Letting go is giving way to another kind of awareness, the power to embrace the world as you are and not get over bored with it.

My PA says that I am discovering another soul that may be better able to cope with my anguish, limitations, hurts and other pains, just because I have got so much joy, love, positive energy running through. Letting go does not mean giving up. Now I can enjoy every single moment of life, in a glory. Miniscule things such as a flower, a dog barking, the caress of the air on my skin, a smile from an unknown person, a little chat that can touch my heart. Music is highly empowering as well: it can touch in many ways; it makes me forget about my little physical self but remember that I am part of the universe.

Writing this autobiography helps me reach within myself, understanding where and why I went wrong or right. There are loads of regrets but also much fun in comprehending my strange path. It gives a sense to my life, confirms what I always felt within, to never give up because you never know what is around the corner. As you know, Carpe Diem – seize the day – is my saying. It is quite the opposite of resignation.

Knowing and accepting all the hindrances helps to check how I should build my future as a responsible adult. Moreover, endorsing all my limitations strangely helps me feel fulfilled with my existence, as I feel quite excited about these challenges. Although inflicted by the imprisonment of an ill body and brain and stuck in the family house, I have the feeling inside I am going to make it. I realised that shagging the world was not fulfilling for me; it was me experiencing my power in the boudoir. I feel sad about shocking and hurting my parents with the dirtiest parts of my life, but I guess they're got used to my dark side or my raving attitude.

Sometimes it's better not to tell parents everything, or they would hide the truth from themselves to avoid too much pain, but I know their love is unconditional anyway. The dirty part of my existence is also a fun story which I am proud of because it did help me to get through the illness; it empowered me to give such pleasure, without hurting anyone, except a few girls and my parents.

Even though showing my intimate ways and drug urges to the world is against the rules of this society, I cannot help being me and I am sorry if I may shock a few people. I wonder if those few could help me anyway. It is part of the bipolar ways to expose oneself to the world. However, you may have noticed that I have not gone through all the kinky details. The less, the better: this is a tool for me to come to an understanding of my life now. It is definitely not a gift to please my family. We are no longer in the nineteenth century where everything weird was hidden and people were all living in a fake way. In our beautiful time, all truth can come out.

Now I feel like an 80-year-old, stuck in a wheelchair; I cannot get out of the house on my own and need two people for all my basic needs. My father is turning 70 but his balance is so much better than mine. However, I feel very safe physically, mentally and affectively. I have discovered an internal strength looking at my life and I am enjoying the awareness of myself and those around me. I am also enjoying the idea that the world may get to know me through my book. Actually, this was probably the main reason why I started this book, to talk to the world! And it is in writing it that I realised how much I needed to understand myself. I also believe that a film can be made from my book, as it was the original wish behind the book. I was telling everyone about the film I was directing myself. It was a good opportunity to talk to beautiful girls and try to attract them as potential actresses in my film. I am still doing this on Facebook. I love Facebook, as I can be all my different selves and talk to the world as well.

Death is a skyline that everyone is watching. I know I am going to die but I cannot put a marker on when. Who can? Everyone knows they are going to die, and therefore should not be scared – it's part of life. This is why we all should make the most of life whilst we are living. I feel that I am a complete survivor, still kicking for life, knowing that it has got a lot of surprises for me. Learning to control and accept myself gives me a reason for my existence and allows me to expect anything, which is quite exciting. Even death will be a surprise! No wish, but just reality, and I am very lucky to have this condition that won't let me feel any pain anyway.

At the end of the day, accepting who you are is the most important thing in life: it makes you feel stabilised with your good self and gives you a clear and strong identity. It helps you point in the right direction, dealing with responsibilities and the unknown. It does not solve all problems, but it helps to face them in peace and harmony and gives back some positive energy. I realise that it is only by accepting yourself that you can find humour on that journey, and get others to start accepting you too.

Addendum

40th birthday messages

Included below are some of the messages that were sent to Charlie on his fortieth birthday from the people he loves and who love him.

– Dearest Charlie!

You know how happy I have been to be the ghost writer of your biovella: it's been such a rewarding experience full of love, learning, healing and creativity for both of us. My wish for your 40th birthday is the birth and healthy growth of your Book … much love for ever. Mab

– Thank you Charlie for letting me be your 'second mother'. I love you. Cleo

– Dearest Charlie

Wishing you a massive happy birthday. With wonderful memories of the Thomas/Bacchus/Wales craziness and how many gorgeous girls you sweet-talked on those boozy weekends!! Such a special person. How could they resist!! So much love, the Jackson family xx

– CB … how can I put into a few short words how much you mean to us all!? You truly are one of the best!! (Shh … don't tell Matt!!) Thank you for bringing so much light, laughter and happiness to our lives – you teach us all to live by your saying – Carpe diem – happy 40th birthday. Lots of love, Beth xX

– Charlie, O Charlie
Please please stay the samey
Lovely young man that you are.

You preside from your chair
With your lush boho hair
The wildest wheeler of London by far.
Charlie, O Charlie,
May you always remainy
This arty and farty and brilly.
May your voice stay this loud
May you never be cowed
May your path avoid being hilly.
Charlie, O Charlie
As you light the birthday flamey
May you sparkle and glitter and glow.
May your grin be this toothy
May your future be smoothy
And may you always just go with the flow.
Helen

– Happy birthday my darling Charlie. I love you my brother. You are a light in my life and the best person I know. So sad not to be with you on your day – looking forward to celebrating middle age with you. All the love in the world – Lucy xxxx

– Happy Birthday to the coolest dude.
Lots of love, Ali and Ed Xxxx

– Dearest Charlie, the man who gave me my first beer, taught me to dance at a Greek disco and will always be a brother to me. Happy birthday wonderful friend. Love, Ben R xxxxx

– Yo B.I.L Carpe Diem Forever! Loads of Love, S

– Darling Charlie
This year is Your Special Year
Your extended family is large and all here
To celebrate with champagne and beer
One who we all want to cheer
And so without further ado
Happy Birthday Charlie
We all love you
Jeanne and David

– Darling Charlie,

You are a full moon, a rising star, a ray of sunshine, a thunderstorm, an everyday force of nature.
We love you so much!
The Laughton family xxxx

– Dear Charlie,

Although during your 40-year ride through life you have encountered some nasty potholes, you always manage to greet everyone with your 150-watt smile which brightens up the lives of all of us who have the pleasure of knowing you.
Enjoy your party and sorry none of us can be with you.
With our love,
Peter and Jane

– Hello Mr Charlie Bacchus,

Happy 30th (+10) birthday! thank you so much for helping me walk through many of my fears (mostly without you even knowing). I have loved every facet of the CB psyche; the cheeky and the vulnerable, the strength and the gentleness, the kisses and the thumps, the smiles and the frowns.... Thank you for letting me have a little peek into your beautiful mind of imagination and thoughts ... what a gorgeous person you are! I look forward to discovering many more!
You are such a special friend and we love you very much.
Big hug, Kate and her clan!

– Happy Birthday Charlie! Thanks for the best Man Hugs over the years. Less stubble next time please;) Laughter conquers all. Love, the Taunton family

– CB, you really are the man to be. You have taught me such a great deal and working together brings back so many happy memories. Chasing ducks on the common to chasing girls along the high street, you manage to make those close to you smile to no end. Let's celebrate your forty fabulous years in classic CB-style ... rum and coke?
Love your pal, Charlie x

– To the one closest to being my older brother,

You're a shining star in my life, and someone I can always depend upon for a kiss, a hug and a smile.

Not everyone can pull off being 40 with such eloquence and grace, but you're doing an amazing job. May you continue to be an inspiration to all around you.
Love you Charlie boy xxx
Anna

– Charlie – You are a courageous – inspirational – and amazingly positive son – you have brought so many fabulous people and much love into our family – and we are so proud of you – never forget how loved you are – love you forever – Mum and Dad – Carpe Diem

– Dearest Charlie, you have a special place in my heart and always will have. We all send you so much love on this important birthday, from Zoe and family
Xxxx

– Hey cous, I want you to know that I love you loads. You are a big part of my life. I always look forward to hanging out with you – if it's tearing around South London keeping everyone on their toes, staying in to play chess or watch a film, and sitting in the garden. I can't wait for the next adventure. Love, Ralph

– Charlie. Your charisma and charm always brings the best out of people and you have taught me a lot over the years. You are an important friend and although you are reaching old age now there is more vibrancy and youth in you than anyone else I know. Stay awesome! Ben

– Happy Happy Birthday Charlie!! I hope you have the best time celebrating with all your friends and family! I'm very much looking forward to future walks on the common & lots of cafe trips! Lots of love from Sally(PA) Xx

– Dear Charlie,

Happy 40th Birthday!!!

Can't believe it is 25 years since you were cajoled into taking your older sister's friend to the sixth-form party. You are and always have been so handsome and such a gent. We had such a nice time, and so many fun times since then. There's been some hilarious moments.
Sending you, lots and lots of love from Laura and Dan x x

– Charlie,
I don't think I fully appreciated the impact it would have when I left London,
I'm not talking about the impact it would have on you, I am talking of the impact it would have on me.
When I first met you I don't think either of us realised the journey we were about to embark on,
The friendship we were about to find, or the memories of laughter and love that we were about to share,
I think they are the best moments in life, the ones that you don't expect to happen, but enrich the soul.
When I think of London, I think of you, when I think of University, I think of you, When I think of football, talking to ladies or drinking hot chocolates (with all the whipped cream) – I think of you,
and even though we aren't together, that we can't see each other daily, I know that you are never far away.
I know that even though physically, I have left London, we will forever keep a piece of each other in our thoughts and in our lives because that's what true friendship is,
realising that friendship isn't a physical measure, something you can weigh or sell, but something that warms you to your core because of the way it has affected your life.
In life, people chase all sorts of things, perhaps we chase things because at the time we perceive them as needs, I don't know.
I do know however, that as time moves on, your perception on these things change too,
When I came to see you each week, I realised that the wants that I had been perceiving as needs sometimes became distorted,
I didn't need to be stressing over exams, I didn't need to be stressing over social media, I didn't need to be stressing over girlfriends,
you had an amazing way of keeping calm, keeping cool, letting lifes worries lift you up instead of drag you down and that my friend,
is one of the most incredible things to be around, your smile, your humour and your devilish personality make you … enriching to be around.
You my friend, you enrich my soul. Never lose that.
Miss you buddy, the brother from the other mother. All my love,
Robin

– A funny little memory of Charlie that has always stuck in my mind…

Tea-time after school at the Bacchus's.

When Hannah cooked us spaghetti she would test if it was cooked by throwing it on to the wall – if it stuck it was ready. One day she threw it too high and it stuck to the ceiling so Charlie, always the show off, climbed up like a monkey onto a chair balanced on the kitchen table to get the piece of spaghetti down with Hannah shouting at him to get down. Charlie grabbed the spaghetti and then jumped from the table on to the kitchen counter and ran round the kitchen with Hannah chasing him. I remember being in fits of giggles and got a little talking to from Hannah that 'laughing at a show-off only encourages them'. But that's why we all love Charlie so much, isn't it? Such a show-off but always so funny and charming with it. Love you my brother from another mother and father x Clare

– Rap to Charlie:
Hello my good friend Charlie
Now bro don't you blame me
'Cos I missed your special birthday
Travelling in the US of A
We go back a long long way
Thru' happy and some difficult days
You played your cards as they lay
Always showing courage and humour yea!
Here's to you bro!!
From Geoff a.k.a. Jeffrey Xx

– Happy birthday, Charlie, and very many congratulations on completing your book! You (and your whole family) have dealt with adversity so very well, and my whole team loved and admired you.
Mike

– Charlie, my dear friend.

It's the big 4–0 and I bet you'd say age is just a number and you'd be right.

But this milestone feels like it's high time to let you know just how important you are to me, to all of us.

You are an inspiration.

To me, to my little son and to everyone who meets you. Your energy, your humour, your zest for life and love for people is astounding.

I am so proud to be know you, to call you one of my best friends. Thank you for truly enriching my life with your beautiful spirit. You are so loved. Catlain xxx

– So very sorry to be missing your big 40 we will raise a glass to you. You are having an incredible and challenging journey in life which you cope with in your family. Your bravery and strength always impressed me and we are proud of you. I have so many fond memories of you as a boy with your football in tow and your wonderful paintings and sketches. Happy birthday day big man; loves you lots. Devon family. XX

– Happy childhood memories, The Bacchus's, and friends.... Scottish Island holiday in the sunshine, freedom on the beautiful beaches and in the sea. All kids together, magical times

Wales and The Bacchus cottage across the valley, beautiful places, wonderful friends, endless weekends and parties, talks, walks and fun with close friends. Crazy times, peaceful times. Growing up together. Happy memories always xx

– Footballing, Artistic Charlie. Talented boy! Gorgeous Charlie, so good looking. Special, Brave, generous Charlie who has always been loving and been loved. Charlie with the biggest heart.
Huge hugs and Happy Happy Birthday with all my love Rachel xxxxxxxx

– Charlie, master of all trades, jack of none. Here's to you and all the good times you bring, your friend,
Max

– Charlie, you're without a doubt the 'Silverest' Silver Tongue Cavalier we know! We love you dearly my friend! Barney, Jack and Tim xx

– Dear Charlie,

I wish you all the best for your 40th celebration.

Since we first met in 1995 many things have happened in your life.

I am deeply impressed by you attitude and spirit, and can only wish you the very best for the future.
Your godfather and friend Jacob

– Message from Layla

To my darling Bro. Look at how many special people you have in your life? You have filled their life with inspiration, laughter, craziness and love. I am so incredibly proud of who you are. You are a beautiful, wise, gentle and loving brother to me and an incredibly special uncle to your niece and nephew. I treasure with every cell in my body the wonderful adventures we had together when we were growing up. The amazing holidays in beautiful places and such happy happy times in Wales with family and friends. The wild teenage party days and the years that have whizzed by so fast since … somehow now decades long! Some days have been really hard, but whatever has happened in our lives, you and I can always make each other laugh and have a strength in our love for each other and our beautiful brother Matt. How lucky we have been darling Bro, to have had a mum and dad who have unconditionally loved us and to have friends and family who have touched our hearts so profoundly. I am always going to be here for you darling Bro. I love you more than the moon. Love Layla

For Product Safety Concerns and Information please contact our EU representative GPSR@taylorandfrancis.com
Taylor & Francis Verlag GmbH, Kaufingerstraße 24, 80331 München, Germany

www.ingramcontent.com/pod-product-compliance
Ingram Content Group UK Ltd.
Pitfield, Milton Keynes, MK11 3LW, UK
UKHW022157190926
475702UK00003B/67
9781138331235